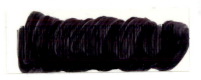

Diagnostic Ultrasound

Diagnostic Ultrasound

STEWART C. BUSHONG, Sc.D., F.A.C.R., F.A.C.M.P.

Professor of Radiologic Science
Department of Radiology
Baylor College of Medicine
Houston, Texas

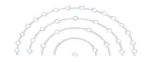

ESSENTIALS OF MEDICAL IMAGING SERIES

McGraw-Hill
Health Professions Division

New York   St. Louis   San Francisco   Auckland   Bogotá   Caracas   Lisbon   London   Madrid
Mexico City   Milan   Montreal   New Delhi   San Juan
Singapore   Sydney   Tokyo   Toronto

McGraw-Hill

*A Division of The **McGraw·Hill** Companies*

DIAGNOSTIC ULTRASOUND

Essentials of Medical Imaging Series

Copyright © 1999 by The McGraw-Hill Companies, Inc. All rights reserved.
Printed in the United States of America. Except as permitted under the
United States Copyright Act of 1976, no part of this publication may be
reproduced or distributed in any form or by any means, or stored in a data
base or retrieval system without the prior written permission of the publisher.

1 2 3 4 5 6 7 8 9 0   MALMAL   9 9

ISBN 0-07-012017-X

This book was set in Berkeley by V&M Graphics.
The editors were John J. Dolan and Peter McCurdy.
The production supervisor was Heather Barry.
The text designer was José R. Fonfrias.
The drawings were created by Robert Lapsley.
The cover designer was Robert Freese.
Malloy Lithographing, Inc. was printer and binder.

This book is printed on acid-free paper.

Visit The McGraw-Hill Health Professions Website at
http://www.mghmedical.com

Cataloging-in-Publication data is on file for this title at the Library of
Congress.

Contents

Preface

IMAGING SCIENCE has changed considerably over the past twenty years. These changes have brought an incredible increase in information, understanding and innovation. One result is that, today, imaging technologists, medical physicists and physicians must know far more than their predecessors. The fund of knowledge required of these health professionals, especially the imaging technologist, for any of the qualifying examinations is so vast that the demands on learning and teaching are considerable.

Accompanying this expansion of knowledge are substantial changes in our occupational opportunities. Limited licensure, cross-training and job splitting are changing the required competence and responsibilities of the imaging technologist. The principal focus of these occupational changes is to obtain more production with fewer employees. Managed healthcare will continue to exert economic and occupational restrictions on the imaging technologist.

This book is one in a series designed to make the learning process easier for the imaging professional. Diagnostic ultrasound imaging is perhaps more widely used today than x ray imaging because it is not restricted to the imaging physician, the radiologist. For example, apparently in excess of seventy percent of all pregnancies are imaged with ultrasound. This volume presents the essential facts of the physics of diagnostic ultrasound imaging. Additional volumes concentrate on other specialty topics and areas of examination.

None of these volumes is a textbook. Sometimes, especially when preparing for an examination, it is easier to commit statements of fact to memory while working with other sources to gain a better understanding of those facts. Each volume contains extensive statements of fact that the author believes are essential for satisfactory completion of the respective qualification examination. These volumes are well illustrated because, as has been said, "A picture is worth a thousand words." Where graphs, charts or tables are included, they are also accompanied with brief statements of fact. At the end of each chapter, there are practice questions patterned after the respective qualification examinations, such as the ABR, the AMBP, ARDMS, the CNMT and especially the ARRT and its subspecialty exams in quality management, mammography, computed tomography, cardiovascular-interventional technology and magnetic resonance imaging. Most examination panels, especially the ARRT, principally use Type A questions: a statement or stem followed by four incorrect answers and one correct answer. Type K questions are used less frequently. These contain multiple statements and the candidate selects the correct combination of answers. The practice questions provided here are of both types.

At the end of each volume, there are four appendices that the student and educator will find particularly helpful. Appendix A is a rather complete glossary of terms employed in imaging science and imaging technology. The student should pay particular attention to this appendix and attempt to know and understand each definition. You will find this very helpful at examination time. Appendix B lists the latest textbook publications covering the respective information areas of the volume. Appendix C contains the answers to the practice questions. Finally, Appendix D, Additional Resources, identifies sources of educational material covering the topics of the book. Here the student will find exceptional literature references to aid in understanding through additional reading of a particular subject. The educator will find this section helpful when assigning special topics or special projects to students.

I am particularly grateful to Yvonne Young and Robert Lapsley. Yvonne was exceptionally helpful with manuscript preparation, not only processing but also editing. Lapsley drew all of the illustrations and was very creative.

Medical imaging as practiced today in all of its forms is based on special principles of physics. To many students, physics is the most feared of subjects—it does not have to be. The purpose of this volume is to ease that learning process, prepare the student for examination and help to make physics fun.

STEWART C. BUSHONG, Sc.D., F.A.C.R., F.A.C.M.P.

The Nature of Diagnostic Ultrasound

- Sound is a **longitudinal mechanical** wave. It is not part of the electromagnetic spectrum.

- Sound is **mechanical** because it requires matter, which is caused to vibrate in wavelike fashion.

- Sound is **longitudinal** because the vibration of molecules in air or tissue is in the direction of the sound.

- In contrast, electromagnetic radiation [e.g., x-ray, light, radio frequency (RF)] is a transverse wave because the associated electric and magnetic fields vary in intensity perpendicular to the direction of radiation.

- Sound is described by its frequency. Expressed in hertz (Hz).

- One hertz is equal to one cycle or wavelength of sound passing each second. 1 Hz = 1 cycle per second.

- Amplitude is the maximum-to-minimum value of the oscillation of a particle or pressure.

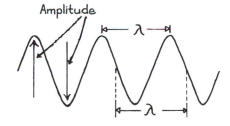

Amplitude

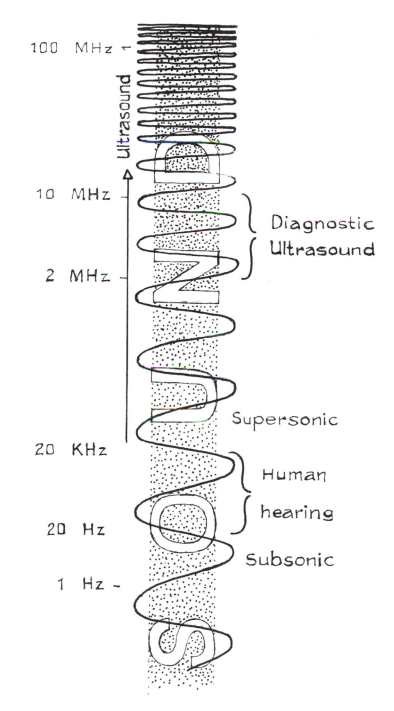

- Sound encompasses the range of frequencies that can be heard by humans, 20 to 20,000 Hz.

- Infrasound lies below the range of human hearing; it is subsonic.

- **Ultrasound** lies above the range of human hearing; it is supersonic.

- Diagnostic ultrasound lies in the range of approximately 1 to 10 megahertz (MHz).

- Ultrasound was first developed for *sound navigation and ranging* (sonar).

Velocity of ultrasound in various materials (m/s)

Biological material		Nonbiological material	
Air	330	Mercury	1450
Fat	1450	Castor oil	1500
Water	1480	PZT	4000
Soft tissue	1540	Steel	5850
Blood	1570		
Muscle	1585		
Bone	4080		

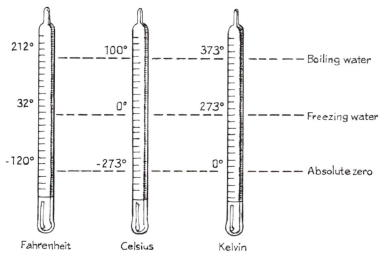

PHYSICAL UNITS OF MEASURE

- **Velocity** is the rate of change of the position of an object—the ultrasound wave—with time.

- The velocity of ultrasound in soft tissue is **1540 m/s.**

- The transit time of ultrasound in soft tissue is 6.5 μs/cm.

- The time from pulse emission to echo reception is 13 μs for each centimeter of depth to reflector.

- **Force** is the push or pull exerted on objects, such as tissue molecules.

- Force equals mass times acceleration. Expressed in newtons (N): $1\ N = 1\ kg\ m/s^2$.

- We express the force of gravity in pounds. $1\ N = 2.2\ lb$.

- **Work** is the force applied to an object, such as a tissue molecule, times the distance over which it is applied.

- Work equals force times distance. Expressed in joules (J): $1\ J = 1\ Nm$.

- **Energy** is the ability to do work. Expressed in joules (J).

- Work and energy are expressed by the same unit, the joule (J).

- **Power** is the rate of doing work on an object.

- Power equals work divided by time. Expressed in watts (W). $1\ W = 1\ J/s$.

- There are two types of energy involved with diagnostic ultrasound: mechanical energy and thermal energy.

- There are two types of **mechanical energy: kinetic energy,** or the energy of motion, and **potential energy,** or the stored energy of position.

- Kinetic energy is imparted to tissue molecules by ultrasound.

- The kinetic energy of tissue molecules results in heat, or **thermal energy.**

- The principal energy transfer between diagnostic ultrasound and tissue causes a temperature rise expressed in degrees centigrade (°C).

- The unit of heat is the calorie (cal). One calorie is the energy necessary to raise the temperature of 1 g of tissue 1°C.

- Energy deposition of approximately 4 J is equivalent to 1 cal, though this will not raise tissue temperature by 1°C because of the body's rapid heat dissipation.

THE WAVE EQUATION

- Unlike x rays, ultrasound requires matter—tissue—in order to travel.

- The movement of an ultrasound wave through tissue or from one tissue to another is called **propagation**.

- Ultrasound is the wave phenomenon consisting of high pressure (**compression**) and low pressure (**rarefaction**) in tissue.

- One **wavelength** (λ) is the distance between adjacent areas of rarefaction or compression.

- Ultrasound obeys the generalized wave equation: velocity (v) equals frequency (f) times wavelength (λ).

- **Frequency** (f) is the number of wavelengths that pass a given point in tissue in one second. Expressed in hertz (Hz).

- **Period** (T) is the time required for one complete wavelength to pass.

- Period and frequency are inversely related.

- Period and wavelength are the same. Period is expressed in time (μs) and wavelength in space (mm).

- Ultrasound **propagation speed** is the scientifically correct terminology; we generally call it ultrasound **velocity**.

- Ultrasound velocity is slow in gas, higher in tissue, and highest in solids.

- This velocity sequence is due principally to **compressibility**, not mass density.

- All ultrasound is transmitted through the same type of tissue at the same velocity even though there may be different frequencies.

- **Mass density** (ρ) is the mass per unit volume of a tissue.

$$v = d/t$$

$$F = ma$$

$$W = Fd$$

$$P = w/t$$

$$P = E/t$$

$$T = 1/f$$

$$f = v/\lambda$$

$$KE = \tfrac{1}{2}mv^2$$

$$P = kg/m^3$$

relative ultrasound velocity

solid > liquid > gas

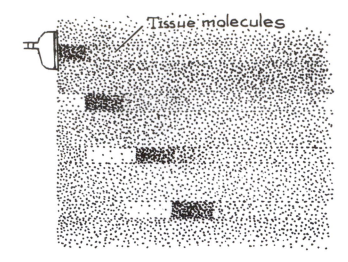

- The velocity of ultrasound is somewhat slower in denser tissue.

COMPRESSIBILITY OF MATTER

- **Compressibility** is the ease with which a volume of tissue can be changed in response to a pressure wave, such as ultrasound.

- Gases are most compressible.

- Solids are least compressible.

- The velocity of the ultrasound is slower in more compressible tissue.

- Ultrasound **phase** refers to the relationship of one wave to another.

- Ultrasound waves whose wavefronts are at the same position are said to be in phase.

- Ultrasound waves whose wavefronts are out of position, one to the other, are said to be out of phase.

- Multiple ultrasound waves can interfere with one another.

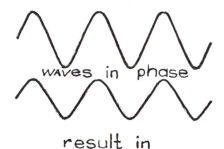

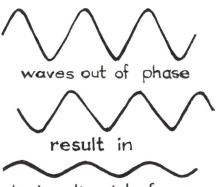

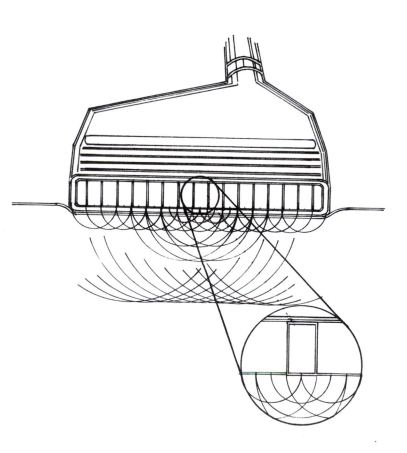

- **Interference** is the interaction of two or more ultrasound beams having different frequency and/or phase.

- **Constructive interference** occurs when ultrasound waves of the same frequency are in phase, resulting in increased amplitude.

- Constructive interference can increase the intensity of an ultrasound beam.

- **Destructive interference** occurs when ultrasound waves are out of phase, resulting in reduced amplitude.

- Destructive interference contributes to ultrasound attenuation.

- The principle of **superposition** is the summation of different ultrasound waves to form a complex wave.

- **Huygens' principle** describes the production of an ultrasound wavefront from individual wavelets.

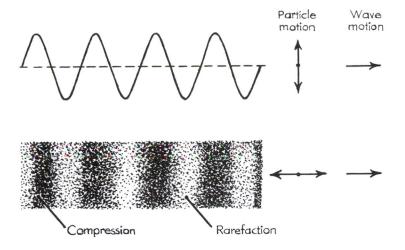

Particle motion / Wave motion

Compression   Rarefaction

Chapter 1 Review Questions

1. **Ultrasonic compression relates to high**

   1. frequency.
   2. pressure.
   3. acoustic velocity.
   4. particle density.

   a. Only 1, 2, and 3 are correct.
   b. Only 1 and 3 are correct.
   c. Only 2 and 4 are correct.
   d. Only 4 is correct.
   e. All are correct.

2. **The wavelength of a 2.25 MHz ultrasound beam is**

   a. 0.15 mm.
   b. 0.7 mm.
   c. 1.5 mm.
   d. 7 mm.
   e. 15 mm.

3. What is the approximate period of a 2.25 MHz ultrasound pulse?
   a. 0.2 μs
   b. 0.4 μs
   c. 2 μs
   d. 4 μs
   e. 20 μs

4. When individual ultrasound waves combine, the process is called
   a. absorption.
   b. attenuation.
   c. interference.
   d. refraction.
   e. dispersion.

5. The conversion of mechanical oscillation to an electrical signal follows
   a. Curie's law.
   b. the Doppler effect.
   c. Snell's law.
   d. the piezoelectric effect.
   e. Huygens' principle.

6. Higher than audible sound, say >20 kHz, is called
   1. infrasound.
   2. supersound.
   3. terasound.
   4. ultrasound.

   a. Only 1, 2, and 3 are correct.
   b. Only 1 and 3 are correct.
   c. Only 2 and 4 are correct.
   d. Only 4 is correct.
   e. All are correct.

7. Approximately how much time passes between pulse transmission and echo reception from a 5 cm deep interface?
   a. 9 μs
   b. 27 μs
   c. 65 μs
   d. 93 μs
   e. 112 μs

8. Rarefaction describes a region of
   a. low pressure.
   b. high pressure.
   c. low velocity.
   d. high velocity.
   e. echogenicity.

9. The frequency of ultrasound is
   a. the inverse of wavelength.
   b. the velocity of particle vibration.
   c. measured in hertz.
   d. the velocity of the wavefront.
   e. determined by the Q value.

10. Ultrasound velocity is faster in tissue of

    a. lower impedance.
    b. lower refractive index.
    c. lower frequency.
    d. higher compressibility.
    e. higher density.

11. What is the approximate velocity of ultrasound in bone?

    a. 300 m/s
    b. 1540 m/s
    c. 4080 m/s
    d. 5550 m/s
    e. 6030 m/s

12. What is the approximate frequency of ultrasound that has a wavelength of 0.4 mm in soft tissue?

    a. 1.7 MHz
    b. 2.2 MHz
    c. 2.9 MHz
    d. 3.8 MHz
    e. 4.2 MHz

13. If the elapsed time between transmission and echo in soft tissue is 39 μs, how deep is the interface?

    a. 2 cm
    b. 3 cm
    c. 5 cm
    d. 7 cm
    e. 9 cm

14. Which of the following is the wave equation?

    a. $v = f\lambda$
    b. $v_t \sin_i = v_i \sin_t$
    c. $\sin_i = 1.22\ \lambda/d$
    d. $Z_i \sin_i = Z_t \sin_t$
    e. $d = \frac{1}{2}\ vt$

15. What is the wavelength of a 2.5 MHz ultrasound beam having velocity of 1520 m/s in soft tissue?

    a. 0.16 mm
    b. 0.62 mm
    c. 1.6 mm
    d. 6.2 mm
    e. 1.6 cm

16. The velocity of ultrasound in soft tissue is approximately

    a. 300 cm/s.
    b. 300 m/s.
    c. 1540 mm/s.
    d. 1540 cm/s.
    e. 1540 m/s.

17. What is the approximate wavelength in soft tissue of a 3 MHz ultrasound beam?

  a. 0.2 mm
  b. 0.5 mm
  c. 2 mm
  d. 5 mm
  e. 2 cm

18. Who among the following stated that positions on a wavefront can be considered point sources for secondary wavelets?

  a. Snell
  b. Doppler
  c. Young
  d. Huygens
  e. Curie

19. A general term to describe an ultrasound wave is

  a. energy.
  b. quadratic.
  c. longitudinal.
  d. matter.
  e. transverse.

20. Which of the following are characteristic of diagnostic ultrasound?

  1. can be transmitted through a vacuum
  2. transverse wave
  3. electromagnetic wave
  4. mechanical vibration wave

  a. Only 1, 2, and 3 are correct.
  b. Only 1 and 3 are correct.
  c. Only 2 and 4 are correct.
  d. Only 4 is correct.
  e. All are correct.

21. Less than audible sound, say < 20 Hz, is called

  1. acoustisonic.
  2. infrasonic.
  3. monosonic.
  4. subsonic.

  a. Only 1, 2, and 3 are correct.
  b. Only 1 and 3 are correct.
  c. Only 2 and 4 are correct.
  d. Only 4 is correct.
  e. All are correct.

22. The conversion of an electrical signal to an oscillating mechanical wave follows

  a. Curie's law.
  b. the Doppler effect.
  c. Snell's law.
  d. the piezoelectric effect.
  e. Huygens' principle.

23. **Which of the following imaging radiations is/are electromagnetic?**

    1. x ray
    2. visible light
    3. radiofrequency
    4. ultrasound

    a. Only 1, 2, and 3 are correct.
    b. Only 1 and 3 are correct.
    c. Only 2 and 4 are correct.
    d. Only 4 is correct.
    e. All are correct.

24. **Ultrasound frequency is expressed in**

    a. hertz (Hz).
    b. mW/cm^2.
    c. mg/cm^3.
    d. newtons (N).
    e. rads.

25. **What can an ultrasound transducer do?**

    1. convert an electrical signal into ultrasound
    2. convert sound into ultrasound
    3. convert ultrasound into an electrical signal
    4. convert ultrasound into sound

    a. Only 1, 2, and 3 are correct.
    b. Only 1 and 3 are correct.
    c. Only 2 and 4 are correct.
    d. Only 4 is correct.
    e. All are correct.

26. **In applying the wave equation, the term period means the**

    a. frequency.
    b. wavelength.
    c. velocity.
    d. time of one cycle.
    e. time of one pulse.

27. **A longitudinal wave is one in which**

    a. the wavelength is shorter than the frequency.
    b. the wavelength is longer than the frequency.
    c. the total energy equals the incremental energy.
    d. the oscillating energy disturbance is in the direction of the wave motion.
    e. the oscillating energy disturbance is perpendicular to the direction of the wave motion.

28. **Slowest to fastest, which of the following properly sequences ultrasound velocity in tissue?**

    a. air, fat, bone, blood, muscle
    b. fat, air, blood, muscle, bone
    c. blood, muscle, fat, air, bone
    d. bone, muscle, fat, blood, air
    e. air, fat, blood, muscle, bone

29. As an ultrasound pulse passes, tissue particles change concentration. Highest concentration is called

    a. ionization.
    b. excitation.
    c. compaction.
    d. compression.
    e. rarefaction.

30. Which of the following characteristics apply to both diagnostic ultrasound and x rays?

    a. both obey the wave equation
    b. velocity and frequency are inversely proportional
    c. matter must be present for transmission
    d. molecular compression and rarefaction occur
    e. interaction via electron excitation

31. Piezo- is derived from the Greek meaning

    a. convert.
    b. energy.
    c. pressure.
    d. transceive.
    e. transduce.

32. Which equation is used to compute wavelength?

    a. $v_i \sin \theta_i = v_t \sin \theta_t$
    b. $v = f\lambda$
    c. $d = \frac{1}{2} vt$
    d. $\sin \theta_i = 1.22 \lambda/d$
    e. $PRF = FR \times LD$

33. Ultrasound is defined as sound having frequency

    a. below 20 Hz.
    b. between 20 Hz and 20 kHz.
    c. above 20 kHz.
    d. between 20 kHz and 1MHz.
    e. between 1 and 5 MHz.

34. Which of the following tissues transmit sound with the highest velocity?

    a. bone
    b. blood
    c. fat
    d. lung
    e. muscle

35. E = energy, d = distance, m = mass and t = time. Which of the following defines power (*P*)?

    a. m/t
    b. m/d
    c. d/t
    d. E/t
    e. E/d

36. **Huygens' principle describes the**

    a. formation of a wavefront.
    b. piezoelectric effect.
    c. attenuation of ultrasound.
    d. reflection of ultrasound.
    e. change in ultrasound velocity at an interface.

37. **Which of the following are acoustic variables?**

    1. mass density
    2. particle motion
    3. pressure
    4. temperature

    a. Only 1, 2, and 3 are correct.
    b. Only 1 and 3 are correct.
    c. Only 2 and 4 are correct.
    d. Only 4 is correct.
    e. All are correct.

38. **Ultrasound velocity in soft tissue is 1540 m/s. Which of the following has velocity closest to soft tissue?**

    a. blood
    b. bone
    c. fat
    d. liver
    e. lung

39. **A transverse wave is one in which**

    a. the wavelength is shorter than the frequency.
    b. the wavelength is longer than the frequency.
    c. the total energy equals the incremental energy.
    d. the oscillating energy disturbance is in the direction of the wave motion.
    e. the oscillating energy disturbance is perpendicular to the direction of the wave motion.

40. **The velocity of ultrasound in tissue depends mainly on**

    a. compressibility.
    b. frequency.
    c. Q value.
    d. mass density.
    e. spatial pulse length (SPL).

41. **The rate at which work is done or energy used is**

    a. duty factor (DF).
    b. Q value.
    c. impedance.
    d. intensity.
    e. power.

42. **Ultrasound waves**
    1. represent mechanical vibrations.
    2. can travel through a vacuum.
    3. transfer energy when traveling through tissue.
    4. are at the low-energy end of the electromagnetic spectrum.

    a. Only 1, 2, and 3 are correct.
    b. Only 1 and 3 are correct.
    c. Only 2 and 4 are correct.
    d. Only 4 is correct.
    e. All are correct.

43. **What is the approximate wavelength range for diagnostic ultrasound?**
    a. 0.1 to 1.0 μm
    b. 1 to 10 μm
    c. 10 to 100 μm
    d. 100 to 1000 μm
    e. 1000 to 10,000 μm

44. **Included in the equation for depth to an interface (the range equation) are**
    a. distance, time, velocity.
    b. distance, wavelength, velocity.
    c. frequency, time, velocity.
    d. reflectivity, time, wavelength.
    e. reflectivity, wavelength, velocity.

45. **What is the approximate wavelength of 2 MHz ultrasound in soft tissue?**
    a. 0.13 μm
    b. 0.8 μm
    c. 1.3 μm
    d. 800 μm
    e. 1300 μm

46. **Approximately how far will sound travel in soft tissue in 10 μs?**
    a. 0.6 mm
    b. 1.5 mm
    c. 6 mm
    d. 15 mm
    e. 60 mm

47. **Which of the following frequencies would include diagnostic ultrasound?**
    1. 10 Hz
    2. 10 kHz
    3. 100 kHz
    4. 10 MHz

    a. Only 1, 2, and 3 are correct.
    b. Only 1 and 3 are correct.
    c. Only 2 and 4 are correct.
    d. Only 4 is correct.
    e. All are correct.

48. Which of the following statements regarding ultrasound velocity is true?
    a. Velocity and frequency remain constant with changes in wavelength.
    b. Velocity is constant regardless of the wavelength.
    c. Velocity increases with increasing frequency.
    d. Velocity decreases with increasing mass density.
    e. Higher optical density suggests higher velocity.

49. As an ultrasound pulse passes, tissue particles change concentration. Lowest concentration is called
    a. ionization.
    b. excitation.
    c. compaction.
    d. compression.
    e. rarefaction.

50. The physical characteristics of audible sound are similar to those of ultrasound, therefore it is true that
    a. velocity is the same in all materials.
    b. velocity depends on its pitch or tone.
    c. as loudness is increased, so will velocity.
    d. the smaller the source, the more collimated the sound.
    e. the higher the frequency, the more collimated the sound.

51. When two ultrasound waves exist simultaneously in the same medium,
    a. they will interfere constructively if traveling in the same direction with the same phase.
    b. they will interfere destructively if of different frequencies.
    c. standing waves will be produced if they are traveling in the same direction with the same phase.
    d. standing waves will be produced if they are traveling in the same direction but out of phase.
    e. beat frequencies result from two very different frequencies.

52. Diagnostic ultrasound resonance occurs
    1. in one-quarter-wavelength piezoelectric crystals.
    2. when reflecting surfaces are separated by a half wavelength.
    3. when reflecting surfaces are separated by any number of half wavelengths.
    4. when destructive interference patterns exist.

    a. Only 1, 2, and 3 are correct.
    b. Only 1 and 3 are correct.
    c. Only 2 and 4 are correct.
    d. Only 4 is correct.
    e. All are correct.

53. Sound emitted with a frequency of 10 Hz would be called
    a. subsonic.
    b. supersonic.
    c. audible.
    d. hyposonic.
    e. hypersonic.

54. **Ultrasound and x rays differ in which of the following ways?**
    1. One is transverse, the other is longitudinal.
    2. One has constant frequency, the other variable frequency.
    3. One has constant velocity, the other variable velocity.
    4. One has constant wavelength, the other variable wavelength.

    a. Only 1, 2, and 3 are correct.
    b. Only 1 and 3 are correct.
    c. Only 2 and 4 are correct.
    d. Only 4 is correct.
    e. All are correct.

55. **In which of the following does ultrasound travel fastest?**
    a. air
    b. bone
    c. steel
    d. soft tissue
    e. fat

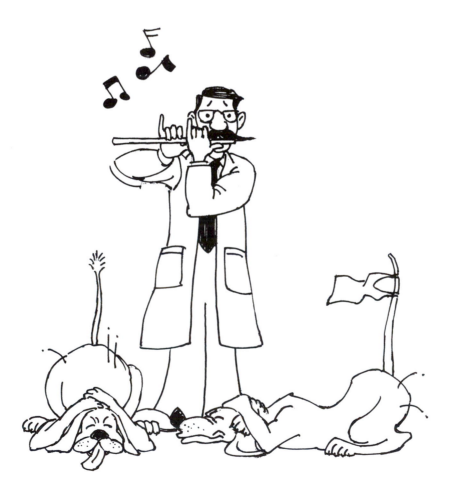

Ultrasound Interaction with Tissue

- X ray images are made from radiation **transmitted** through the body.

- Nuclear medicine and magnetic resonance images depend on radiation **emitted** by the body.

- Ultrasound images are made from radiation **reflected** within the body.

- **Attenuation** is the reduction in the intensity of an ultrasound beam as it travels through tissue.

- Attenuation is the result of several independent, different interactions of the ultrasound beam with tissue: absorption, scattering, reflection, refraction, diffraction, interference and beam divergence.

- The degree of attenuation of a homogenous tissue is expressed by the attenuation coefficient ($\propto$).

- The ultrasound attenuation coefficient is expressed in dB/cm/MHz.

- As frequency is increased, the attenuation coefficient is increased proportionally.

attenuation —
- absorption
- scattering
- reflection
- refraction
- diffraction
- interference
- divergence

$$\text{attenuation} = \text{frequency} \times \text{attenuation coefficient} \times \text{tissue path}$$
$$(dB) = (MHz) \quad (dB/cm/MHz) \quad (cm)$$

- In soft tissue, the attenuation coefficient is equal to approximately 1 dB/cm/MHz.

ABSORPTION

- **Absorption** results from the internal friction created by the vibration of tissue molecules.

- Absorption is normally the highest component of attenuation.

- Absorption is the conversion of the energy of the ultrasound beam to heat.

Attenuation coefficient at 1 MHz

Material	α (dB/cm)
Lung	41
Bone	20
Air	12
Soft tissue	1.0
Fat	.63
Blood	.18
Water	.0022

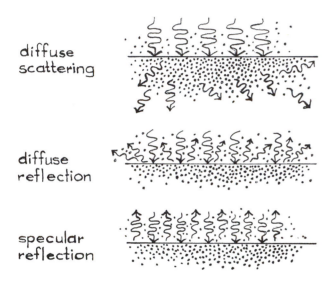

diffuse scattering

diffuse reflection

specular reflection

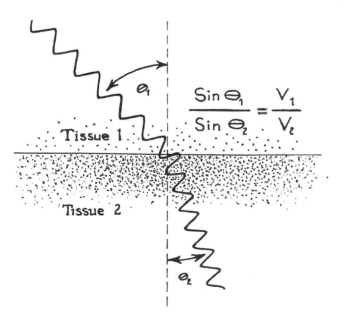

$$\frac{\sin \theta_1}{\sin \theta_2} = \frac{V_1}{V_2}$$

- Absorption is the **only** process that directly removes energy from the ultrasound beam.

- The loss of energy through absorption results in tissue heating.

- **Viscosity** is the degree to which a fluid resists flow.

- Water and blood have low viscosity. Muscle and fat have high viscosity.

- High viscosity results in increased absorption.

- **Relaxation time** is the time required for a tissue molecule to return to its original position after an ultrasound wave passes.

- Tissues with long relaxation times absorb more ultrasound energy.

- Ultrasound absorption resulting from tissue viscosity and relaxation time are affected by frequency.

- Higher frequency results in increased ultrasound absorption.

SCATTERING

- **Scattering** results when the ultrasound beam in a homogenous tissue is dispersed by interactions with individual molecules.

- Scattering at a tissue interface is called **backscatter**.

- Scattering from a smooth mirror-like tissue interface is called **specular** reflection.

- Specular reflectors are the diaphragm, liver, and gallbladder.

- Specular reflection is most useful for imaging.

- Scattering from an irregular tissue interface is called diffuse or nonspecular reflection and results in increased ultrasound attenuation.

- Diffuse reflection occurs, for example, at red blood cells and liver parenchyma.

- Diffuse reflection accounts for most ultrasound echoes used to make an image.

- **Refraction** is the change in direction of ultrasound as it crosses a tissue interface.

- Refraction can also be considered a scattering process.

- Refraction of ultrasound follows **Snell's law**.

- Refraction artifacts are objects or shapes that are not portrayed on the image in their true position.

- **Diffraction** is the uniform spreading of an ultrasound beam as it propagates from the source.

- The smaller the source of ultrasound, the higher the diffraction of the beam.

- Ultrasound diffraction can also occur when passing through a tissue aperture.

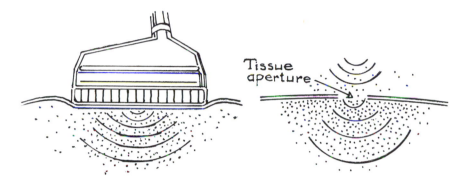

- Diffraction can be considered an additional type of scattering.

- The more an ultrasound beam is diffracted, the more it will be attenuated.

REFLECTION

- A **reflection** is the tissue interaction used to make an image.

- Best reflection occurs from a smooth tissue interface and is called **specular reflection**.

- Examples of tissue specular reflectors are diaphragm, portal vein, renal capsule, and bladder wall.

- Best specular reflection occurs when the ultrasound beam is **perpendicular** to the tissue interface.

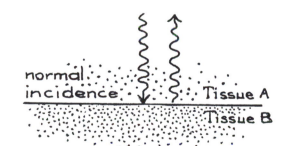

- The term **normal** is often used for perpendicular; they mean the same.

- If an ultrasound beam is not perpendicular to an interface, it is obliquely incident on that interface.

- With oblique incidence, the transmitted beam obeys Snell's law.

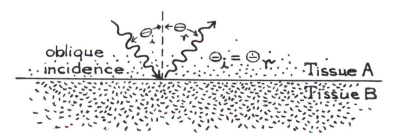

Material	Acoustic impedance (Rayls)
Air	0.0004
Fat	1.38
Oil	1.43
Water	1.48
Amniotic Fluid	1.51
Brain	1.58
Blood	1.61
Kidney	1.62
Liver	1.65
Muscle	1.70
Bone	7.80

$$Z = \rho v$$

$$rayl = (kg/m^3)(m/s)$$

$$= kg/m^2 s$$

- When reflected ultrasound arrives back at the transducer, it is called an **echo**.

- The law of reflection states that the angle of incidence is equal to the angle of reflection from a tissue interface.

- The angle of incidence, θ_i, and the angle of reflection, θ_r, are measured from the perpendicular to the interface, not the interface itself.

- To form an image, the angle of incidence on a tissue interface must not exceed 3°.

- As the angle of incidence increases, so does the angle of reflection, which can result in no echo being received by the transducer.

- The amount of ultrasound reflected at a specular tissue interface is determined by the **acoustic impedance** of each tissue.

- Acoustic impedance (Z) of a tissue is the product of the velocity (v) of ultrasound in that tissue and its mass density (ρ).

- Acoustic impedance (Z) of a tissue is approximately proportional to tissue compressibility, thus low to intermediate in soft tissue, high in bone.

- Acoustic intensity is measured in rayls.

- Tissues having similar acoustic impedance and forming an interface will reflect very little ultrasound. Most is transmitted across the interface.

- Tissues having very different acoustic impedance will reflect a high percentage of ultrasound from a specular reflector. Little will be transmitted.

- Reflectivity, therefore, is determined by tissue acoustic impedance (Z) and the structure of the interface, i.e., specular or diffuse.

Chapter 2 Review Questions

1. Calculate the acoustic impedance of a 2.25 MHz beam in soft tissue.

   a. 0.15 rayl
   b. 0.7 rayl
   c. 1.5 rayl
   d. 7 rayl
   e. 15 rayl

2. What is the approximate mass density of soft tissue?

   1. $10 \ g/cm^3$ 3. $10^6 \ g/m^3$
   2. $1000 \ kg/m^3$ 4. $1 \ g/cm^3$

   a. Only 1, 2, and 3 are correct.
   b. Only 1 and 3 are correct.
   c. Only 2 and 4 are correct.
   d. Only 4 is correct.
   e. All are correct.

3. What approximate percent of a 2.25 MHz ultrasound beam will be reflected from a fat (Z = 1.38 rayl) / muscle (Z = 1.7 rayl) interface?

   a. 1
   b. 5
   c. 10
   d. 30
   e. 50

4. What causes reflection at a tissue interface?

   a. absorption
   b. attenuation
   c. impedance change
   d. velocity change
   e. frequency change

5. Specular reflection occurs only

   a. at high frequency.
   b. at a smooth interface.
   c. with real-time ultrasound.
   d. at a high-impedance interface.
   e. with a focused beam.

6. The change in direction of an ultrasound beam across a tissue interface is due principally to

   a. attenuation.
   b. diffraction.
   c. interference.
   d. reflection.
   e. dispersion.

7. What happens when ultrasound passes from a medium of low acoustic velocity to one of high acoustic velocity?

    a. frequency decreases
    b. frequency increases
    c. wavelength decreases
    d. wavelength increases
    e. velocity increases

8. The coefficient of attenuation of diagnostic ultrasound is approximately

    a. 0.1 dB/cm/MHz.
    b. 1.0 dB/cm/MHz.
    c. 10 dB/cm/MHz.
    d. 100 dB/cm/MHz.
    e. 1000 dB/cm/MHz.

9. Which of the following has highest acoustic attenuation?

    a. bone
    b. fat
    c. kidney
    d. lung
    e. blood

10. The reflection of light from frosted glass is called

    a. diffuse.
    b. refractive.
    c. scattered.
    d. specular.
    e. nonspecular.

11. What happens to ultrasound frequency when a pulse moves from tissue with high acoustic impedance to tissue with low acoustic impedance?

    a. it gets lower
    b. it does not change
    c. it gets higher
    d. it varies
    e. need more information

12. Which of the following most influences the resistance of tissue to ultrasound propagation?

    a. compressibility
    b. mass density
    c. acoustic impedance
    d. index of refraction
    e. dispersion

13. Ultrasound reflected from a rough tissue interface is

    a. called specular reflection.
    b. called diffuse reflection.
    c. refracted.
    d. diffracted.
    e. dispersed.

14. **Acoustic impedance is affected by**

    1. velocity in tissue.
    2. elasticity of tissue.
    3. mass density of tissue.
    4. ultrasound frequency.

    a. Only 1, 2, and 3 are correct.
    b. Only 1 and 3 are correct.
    c. Only 2 and 4 are correct.
    d. Only 4 is correct.
    e. All are correct.

15. **Which of the following is Snell's law?**

    a. $v_i \sin \theta_i = v_t \sin \theta_t$
    b. $v = f\lambda$
    c. $\sin \theta_i = 1.22 \, \lambda/d$
    d. $Z_i \sin \theta_i = Z_t \sin \theta_t$
    e. $d = \frac{1}{2} \, vt$

16. **What is it called when ultrasound diverges through a small aperture?**

    a. absorption
    b. refraction
    c. diffraction
    d. interference
    e. dispersion

17. **Attenuation of ultrasound is dependent on**

    1. frequency.
    2. velocity.
    3. wavelength.
    4. mass density.

    a. Only 1, 2, and 3 are correct.
    b. Only 1 and 3 are correct.
    c. Only 2 and 4 are correct.
    d. Only 4 is correct.
    e. All are correct.

18. **Why does an ultrasonographer apply gel to a patient's skin during imaging?**

    a. to reduce friction
    b. to remove air
    c. to prevent ringdown
    d. to soften skin
    e. to improve reflections

19. **The ultrasonographer should avoid lung because of**

    a. refraction.
    b. reflection.
    c. attenuation.
    d. scattering.
    e. velocity.

20. **When the intensity of a pulse echo is −15 dB, what is the ratio of transmitted to reflected ultrasound?**

    a. 12:1
    b. 16:1
    c. 20:1
    d. 24:1
    e. 32:1

21. Which of the following is a diffuse reflector?

    a. liver
    b. spleen
    c. red blood cells
    d. diaphragm
    e. bone

22. A 2.5 MHz pulse returns from a 3 cm deep interface in the abdomen. Approximately, how much has it been attenuated?

    a. 2.5 dB
    b. 5 dB
    c. 7.5 dB
    d. 10 dB
    e. 15 dB

23. The impedance of tissue A is 0.3 rayl and that of tissue B is 0.6 rayl. What percentage of a beam incident on this interface will be reflected?

    a. <1
    b. 3
    c. 6
    d. 9
    e. 15

24. Which factor determines the amount of ultrasound reflected at an interface?

    a. absorption
    b. attenuation
    c. diffraction
    d. impedance
    e. refraction

25. Which of the following can occur at a tissue interface?

    1. refraction   3. reflection
    2. diffraction   4. absorption

    a. Only 1, 2, and 3 are correct.
    b. Only 1 and 3 are correct.
    c. Only 2 and 4 are correct.
    d. Only 4 is correct.
    e. All are correct.

26. What causes refraction at a tissue interface?

    a. absorption
    b. attenuation
    c. impedance change
    d. velocity change
    e. frequency change

27. What approximate percent of a 5 MHz ultrasound beam will be transmitted through a fat (Z = 1.38 rayl) / muscle (Z = 1.7 rayl) interface?

    a. 10
    b. 25
    c. 50
    d. 75
    e. 99

28. The reflection in a mirror is called
    a. diffuse.
    b. refractive.
    c. scattered.
    d. specular.
    e. nonspecular.

29. Which of the following has lowest acoustic attenuation?
    a. bone
    b. fat
    c. kidney
    d. lung
    e. blood

30. Specular reflection of ultrasound occurs at a
    a. smooth tissue interface.
    b. rough tissue interface.
    c. small tissue interface.
    d. large tissue interface.
    e. homogenous tissue interface.

31. The precise definition of specular reflection requires that
    a. the two tissues have very different ultrasound impedance.
    b. the two tissues have similar ultrasound impedance.
    c. the roughness of the tissue interface be smaller than the ultrasound wavelength.
    d. the roughness of the tissue interface be equal to the ultrasound wavelength.
    e. the roughness of the tissue interface be larger than the ultrasound wavelength.

32. Which tissue has least ultrasound attenuation?
    a. air
    b. blood
    c. bone
    d. fat
    e. muscle

33. Which equation is used to compute the degree of reflection?

    a. $Z = \rho v$ b. $v = \lambda f$ c. $dB = 10 \log \dfrac{I_t}{I_o}$

    d. $\dfrac{\sin_i}{\sin_r} = \dfrac{v_i}{v_r}$ e. $\left(\dfrac{Z_2 - Z_1}{Z_2 + Z_1} \right)^2$

34. Acoustic impedance is the
    a. sum of tissue density and ultrasound velocity.
    b. difference between tissue density and ultrasound velocity.
    c. product of tissue density and ultrasound velocity.
    d. product of tissue density and tissue absorption.
    e. product of tissue density and tissue attenuation.

35. Which of the following contributes to attenuation of an ultrasound beam?

    1. absorption   3. scattering
    2. divergence   4. reflection

    a. Only 1, 2, and 3 are correct.
    b. Only 1 and 3 are correct.
    c. Only 2 and 4 are correct.
    d. Only 4 is correct.
    e. All are correct.

36. Ultrasound reflected from a smooth tissue interface is

    a. called specular reflection.
    b. called diffuse reflection.
    c. refracted.
    d. diffracted.
    e. dispersed.

37. Acoustic impedance is expressed in

    a. hertz (Hz).
    b. mW/cm^2.
    c. dB.
    d. rayl.
    e. joule (J).

38. What is the approximate percent reflection between lung and muscle?

    a. 1
    b. 10
    c. 25
    d. 50
    e. 100

39. Hyperechoic tissue is also

    a. anechoic.
    b. echo-free.
    c. echogenic.
    d. hypersonic.
    e. hyposonic.

40. If the angle of incidence at an interface is greater than the critical angle,

    a. frequency and reflection will increase.
    b. frequency and reflection will decrease.
    c. there will be no frequency change, 100% absorption.
    d. there will be no frequency change, 100% reflection.
    e. there will be no frequency change, 100% transmission.

41. Intrinsic tissue characteristics determine ultrasound

    1. frequency.   3. intensity.
    2. velocity.   4. impedance.

    a. Only 1, 2, and 3 are correct.
    b. Only 1 and 3 are correct.
    c. Only 2 and 4 are correct.
    d. Only 4 is correct.
    e. All are correct.

42. Total reflection occurs at greater than the

    a. reflection angle.
    b. diffraction angle.
    c. refraction angle.
    d. critical angle.
    e. specular angle.

43. What is the approximate attenuation coefficient of 5 MHz ultrasound in soft tissue?

    a. 0.5 dB/cm
    b. 1 dB/cm
    c. 2 dB/cm
    d. 5 dB/cm
    e. 10 dB/cm

44. The ultrasound energy reflected at a tissue interface depends principally on what property of the tissue or ultrasound wave?

    a. attenuation coefficient
    b. beam shape
    c. frequency
    d. impedance
    e. intensity

45. Lowest to highest, arrange the following types of tissue according to acoustic impedance.

    a. gas, liquid, solid
    b. liquid, solid, gas
    c. solid, gas, liquid
    d. liquid, gas, solid
    e. solid, liquid, gas

46. Which property is important in determining the value of acoustic impedance?

    1. mass density   3. velocity
    2. optical density   4. frequency

    a. Only 1, 2, and 3 are correct.
    b. Only 1 and 3 are correct.
    c. Only 2 and 4 are correct.
    d. Only 4 is correct.
    e. All are correct.

47. The product of tissue mass density and velocity is

    a. duty factor (DF).
    b. Q value.
    c. impedance.
    d. intensity.
    e. power.

48. It takes 30 μs for a pulse to travel to an interface and return as an echo. Approximately, how deep is the interface?

    a. <1 cm
    b. 1 cm
    c. 2 cm
    d. 4 cm
    e. 6 cm

49. The reduction in intensity of sound as it penetrates tissue is called

    a. attenuation.
    b. broadening.
    c. damping.
    d. impedance.
    e. specularity.

50. Specular reflections

    1. produce maximum scattering.
    2. require interface irregularities larger than ultrasound wavelength.
    3. require 90° incidence of the transmitted beam.
    4. occur at smooth interfaces.

    a. Only 1, 2, and 3 are correct.
    b. Only 1 and 3 are correct.
    c. Only 2 and 4 are correct.
    d. Only 4 is correct.
    e. All are correct.

51. Anechoic tissue is also

    a. echo-free.
    b. echogenic.
    c. hyperechoic.
    d. hypoechoic.
    e. hyposonic.

52. What is the approximate percent reflection between fat and muscle?

    a. 1
    b. 10
    c. 25
    d. 50
    e. 100

53. Ultrasound absorption increases with increasing

    1. distance in tissue.   3. viscosity.
    2. frequency.   4. molecular relaxation time.

    a. Only 1, 2, and 3 are correct.
    b. Only 1 and 3 are correct.
    c. Only 2 and 4 are correct.
    d. Only 4 is correct.
    e. All are correct.

54. A difference of tissue impedance at an interface will cause

    a. attenuation.

    b. diffraction.

    c. reflection.

    d. refraction.

    e. scattering.

55. Acoustic reflectivity (R)

    a. is equal to density times velocity.

    b. equals 100 if $Z_1 = Z_2$.

    c. is higher for an air/soft tissue interface than for a bone/soft tissue interface.

    d. increases with increasing frequency.

    e. increases with larger wavelength.

56. An ultrasound beam that is perpendicularly incident on a tissue interface will **not** experience

    a. absorption.

    b. attenuation.

    c. diffraction.

    d. reflection.

    e. refraction.

57. During pulse echo (PE) imaging at 5 MHz, 3 cm of tissue will attenuate the beam.

    a. 0.6 dB

    b. 1.7 dB

    c. 3 dB

    d. 5 dB

    e. 15 dB

58. If the angle of incidence at a tissue interface is 90°,

    a. diffraction will not occur.

    b. reflection will not occur.

    c. refraction will not occur.

    d. velocity will not change.

    e. wavelength will not change.

59. The magnitude of the refractive angle can be computed from

    a. Curie's law.

    b. the Doppler effect.

    c. Huygens' principle.

    d. the piezoelectric effect.

    e. Snell's law.

60. The approximate percentage of ultrasound reflected at a lung/soft tissue interface is

    a. <10.

    b. 25.

    c. 50.

    d. 75.

    e. >90.

61. The critical angle of an ultrasound beam on a tissue interface is
    a. usually less than 5°.
    b. approximately 10°.
    c. approximately 25°.
    d. totally transmitting.
    e. dependent on velocity in each tissue.

62. High-frequency transducers have
    a. better resolution and less penetration.
    b. better resolution and more penetration.
    c. reduced resolution and higher intensity.
    d. reduced resolution and less penetration.
    e. reduced resolution and more penetration.

63. As ultrasound is transmitted through tissue, its intensity is reduced by all except
    a. excitation.
    b. absorption.
    c. scattering.
    d. divergence.
    e. diffraction.

64. When a diagnostic ultrasound beam is incident on a tissue interface,
    a. none of the beam will be transmitted.
    b. none of the beam will be reflected.
    c. reflection can occur only when the beam is at right angles to the interface.
    d. maximum reflection occurs at the critical angle.
    e. maximum transmission occurs at the critical angle.

65. When an acoustic wave is transmitted through soft tissue,
    1. intensity is constant.
    2. energy is transferred by Compton scattering.
    3. energy is transferred by electronic excitation.
    4. attenuation occurs.

    a. Only 1, 2, and 3 are correct.
    b. Only 1 and 3 are correct.
    c. Only 2 and 4 are correct.
    d. Only 4 is correct.
    e. All are correct.

66. When a transmitted ultrasound beam changes direction while passing from one medium to another, this is called
    a. reflection.
    b. diffraction.
    c. refraction.
    d. scattering.
    e. attenuation.

67. Acoustic reflectivity (R) is expressed by which of the following?

a. $R = \left(\dfrac{Z_1 \times Z_2}{Z_1 + Z_2}\right)$
b. $R = \left(\dfrac{Z_1 \times Z_2}{Z_1 + Z_2}\right)^2$
c. $R = \dfrac{Z_1 - Z_2}{Z_1 + Z_2}$

d. $R = \left(\dfrac{Z_1 - Z_2}{Z_1 + Z_2}\right)^2$
e. $R = \left(\dfrac{Z_1 \times Z_2}{Z_1 - Z_2}\right)^2$

68. A difference of ultrasound velocity at an interface will cause

a. attenuation.
b. diffraction.
c. reflection.
d. refraction.
e. scattering.

69. The rayl has dimensions of

a. $kg\ m^{-2}s^{-1}$.
b. $kg\ m^{-3}s^{-1}$.
c. $kg\ m^{-3}s^{-2}$.
d. $kg\ m^{-3}$.
e. $kg\ m^{2}s^{-1}$.

70. What is the approximate percent reflectivity (%R) at a blood-brain interface if the acoustic impedance of blood is 1.61×10^6 rayl and that of brain is 1.58×10^6 rayl?

a. 0.00009%
b. 0.009%
c. 0.09%
d. 0.9%
e. 9%

71. The approximate percentage of ultrasound transmitted across a lung/soft tissue interface is

a. <10.
b. 25.
c. 50.
d. 75.
e. >90.

72. Reflections from a smooth tissue interface are called

a. backscatter.
b. diffuse.
c. isotropic.
d. multiple.
e. specular.

73. **Ultrasound attenuation occurs because of**

    1. divergence.   3. absorption.
    2. scattering.   4. refraction.

    a. Only 1, 2, and 3 are correct.
    b. Only 1 and 3 are correct.
    c. Only 2 and 4 are correct.
    d. Only 4 is correct.
    e. All are correct.

74. **Which of the following tissues will attenuate ultrasound the most?**

    a. lung
    b. fat
    c. muscle
    d. bone
    e. blood

75. **Ultrasound pulses are**

    a. poorly transmitted by liquids.
    b. poorly transmitted by solids.
    c. partially reflected at interfaces between two liquids.
    d. totally transmitted at interfaces between two liquids.
    e. totally reflected at a gas liquid interface.

Ultrasound Power and Intensity

- **Energy** is the ability to do work, measured in joules (J).

- **Work** is the result of energy applied, and it too is measured in joules (J).

- **Power** is the rate of doing work measured in watts (W). 1 W = 1 J/s.

- A rock concert releases approximately 100 W of acoustic power, about the same as a light bulb.

- An ultrasound transducer emits acoustic power in the milliwatt (mW) range.

- **Ultrasound intensity** is the preferred measure of the ultrasound beam, not ultrasound power.

- When applied to audible sound, power and intensity are **loudness**.

ACOUSTIC INTENSITY

- Ultrasound intensity is the power that passes through a tissue, expressed in mW/cm^2.

- As ultrasound intensity is increased, the pressure and displacement of tissue molecules increases.

- Ultrasound **amplitude**, although rarely used, is another measure of the ultrasound beam.

- Amplitude is the difference between the maximum and minimum values of either a molecule's displacement, pressure, or velocity.

- Ultrasound intensity is proportional to the amplitude squared. We usually express ultrasound intensity in decibels (dB), which is a relative value.

- Silence is 0 dB compared with conversational speech, which is approximately 60 dB.

Kinetic energy
$$E = \tfrac{1}{2}\, mv^2$$

Potential Energy
$$E = mgh$$

Electromagnetic Energy
$$E = hf$$

Relativistic Energy
$$E = mc^2$$

$$\text{work} = \text{force} \times \text{distance} \ (\text{Joule})$$
$$\text{power} = \text{work}/\text{time} \ (\text{watt})$$
$$\text{intensity} = \text{power}/\text{area} \ (\text{watt}/m^2)$$

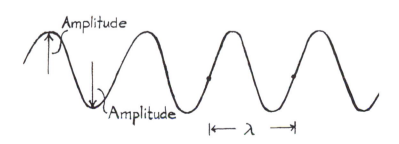

$$\text{decibel (dB)} = 10 \log \frac{\text{reflected intensity}}{\text{emitted intensity}}$$

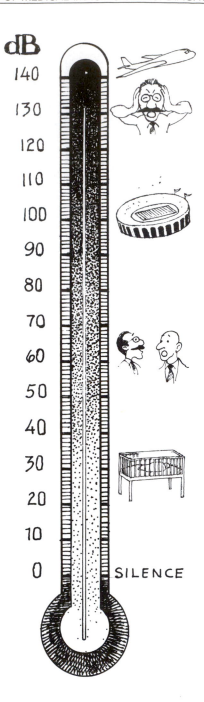

- 1 dB is the smallest difference in loudness that a human ear can distinguish.

- 1 dB equals 10 times the log I/I_o.

- Ultrasound echoes are measured in negative decibels.

- Ultrasound echoes are much lower in intensity than that which was emitted by the transducer.

- −3 dB describes an ultrasound beam with half the intensity of the transmitted beam.

- −10 dB describes an ultrasound beam with only 10% of the transmitted intensity.

- −20 dB describes the ultrasound beam with only 1% of the transmitted intensity.

SPATIAL–TEMPORAL–PULSE: PEAK-AVERAGE

- The intensity of both a continuous-wave (CW) and a pulse echo (PE) ultrasound beam varies in space and time.

- When spatial and temporal intensities are considered, six combinations result: SPTP (highest), SATP-SPTA-SATA (lowest), SAPA-SPPA.

- The **spatial peak** intensity (SP) is greatest along the central axis of the ultrasound beam and at the focal depth of the ultrasound beam.

- The **spatial average** intensity (SA) is <5% of the SP.

- The **temporal peak** intensity (TP) is the maximum intensity present in the ultrasound beam.

- The **temporal average** intensity (TA) takes into account the time during pulse echo ultrasound that no ultrasound is emitted.

interface	approximate echo
soft tissue/gas	0 dB
soft tissue/bone	-20 dB
fat/muscle	-40 dB
liver/spleen	-60 dB

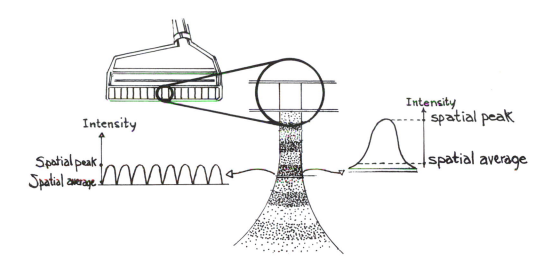

- The **pulse average** intensity (PA) is the average intensity of the several cycles contained within one pulse of ultrasound.

- **Beam uniformity ratio** (BUR) is a measure of the intensity variation of an ultrasound beam.

- The time during pulse echo ultrasound between pulses when no ultrasound is emitted is called the **dead time**.

- The four intensities of importance are: SATA, SPTA, SAPA, and SPPA.

- SATA intensity is the lowest of these four.

- SPPA intensity is the highest of these four.

$$BUR = SP/SA$$

$$DF = TA/PA$$

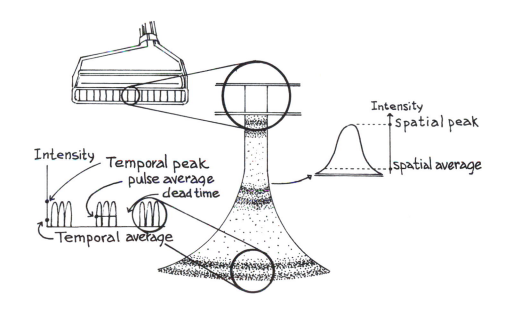

Chapter 3 Review Questions

1. Ultrasound intensity is expressed in
   a. N.
   b. N/cm^2.
   c. mW.
   d. mW/cm^2.
   e. mW/cm^3.

2. Which of the following measures of pulse echo (PE) intensity is highest?
   a. spatial average, temporal average (SATA)
   b. spatial average, temporal peak (SATP)
   c. spatial peak, temporal average (SPTA)
   d. spatial peak, temporal peak (SPTP)
   e. spatial peak, pulse average (SPPA)

3. What is the approximate intensity of a 2 MHz ultrasound beam reflected from a soft tissue/bone interface?
   a. −1 dB
   b. −2 dB
   c. −3 dB
   d. −4 dB
   e. −5 dB

4. What is the approximate intensity of a 2 MHz ultrasound beam reflected from a soft tissue/bone interface at a depth of 3 cm in soft tissue?
   a. −3 dB
   b. −5 dB
   c. −9 dB
   d. −12 dB
   e. −16 dB

5. When applied to diagnostic ultrasound, dynamic range means
   a. frequency bandwidth.
   b. frequency range of transducer.
   c. range of detectable signal intensities.
   d. pulse repetition.
   e. spatial resolution.

6. What is the equivalent to one-half value layer attenuation?
   a. −0.5 dB
   b. −1.0 dB
   c. −3 dB
   d. −5 dB
   e. −10 dB

7. The decibel is a unit used to describe what feature of an ultrasound beam?
   a. absorption
   b. attenuation
   c. impedance
   d. intensity
   e. refractivity

8. Why is beam intensity usually maximum at the focal length?
    a. enhancement effects
    b. diffraction effects
    c. refraction effects
    d. shorter spatial pulse length (SPL)
    e. smaller beam diameter

9. When an echo is 20 dB less intense than the transmitted pulse, what fraction of transmitted pulse is it?
    a. 1/10
    b. 1/20
    c. 1/100
    d. 1/200
    e. 1/1000

10. Ultrasound attenuation includes
    1. absorption.   3. scattering.
    2. reflection.   4. reverberation.

    a. Only 1, 2, and 3 are correct.
    b. Only 1 and 3 are correct.
    c. Only 2 and 4 are correct.
    d. Only 4 is correct.
    e. All are correct.

11. Ultrasound attenuation is expressed in
    a. dB.
    b. hertz (Hz).
    c. mW/cm^2.
    d. %.
    e. rayl.

12. Which equation is used to compute acoustic impedance?

    a. $Z = \rho v$ b. $v = \lambda f$ c. $dB = 10 \log \dfrac{I_t}{I_o}$

    d. $\dfrac{\sin_i}{\sin_r} = \dfrac{v_i}{v_r}$ e. $\left(\dfrac{Z_2 - Z_1}{Z_2 + Z_1}\right)^2$

13. Diagnostic ultrasound is sound having frequency
    a. below 20 Hz.
    b. between 20 Hz and 20 kHz.
    c. above 20 kHz.
    d. between 20 kHz and 1 MHz.
    e. between 1-5 MHz.

14. Which of the following measures of pulse echo (PE) intensity is lowest?
    a. spatial average, temporal average (SATA)
    b. spatial average, temporal peak (SATP)
    c. spatial peak, temporal average (SPTA)
    d. spatial peak, temporal peak (SPTP)
    e. spatial peak, pulse average (SPPA)

15. Ultrasound power is expressed in
    a. N.
    b. N/cm^2.
    c. W.
    d. W/cm^2.
    e. W/cm^3.

16. A hydrophone is used principally to measure ultrasound
    a. duty factor (DF).
    b. frequency.
    c. intensity.
    d. Q value.
    e. wavelength.

17. An amplifier increases the echo signal by $\times 1000$. Its amplification gain is
    a. 10 dB.
    b. 20 dB.
    c. 30 dB.
    d. 100 dB.
    e. 1000 dB.

18 Amplification gain is set at 32 dB. If the gain is reduced by a half, the new gain will be
    a. 8 dB.
    b. 16 dB.
    c. 24 dB.
    d. 29 dB.
    e. 31 dB.

19. When tissue is exposed to ultrasound,
    a. the unit of intensity is mW/cm^2.
    b. the unit of ultrasound dose is the rad.
    c. the unit of ultrasound dose is the decibel (dB).
    d. if a beam has a 30 dB gain, that means it is 30% more intense.
    e. if the reflected beam is -40 dB, it is only 0.1% of the transmitted beam.

20. Which of the following is equivalent to increasing signal intensity by 10 times?
    a. 1 dB
    b. 3 dB
    c. 5 dB
    d. 10 dB
    e. 20 dB

21. Spatial average, temporal average (SATA) ultrasound is measured in
    a. dB.
    b. dB/cm.
    c. dB/cm/MHz.
    d. mW.
    e. mW/cm^2.

22. Diagnostic ultrasound intensity is measured in
    a. watts (W).
    b. W/cm^2.
    c. rad.
    d. gray.
    e. decibels (dB).

23. If the intensity of ultrasound beam A is compared with that of beam B, its value in decibels will be
    a. $10\ e^{-\mu x}$.
    b. 10 In (A/B).
    c. 10 log (A/B).
    d. 10 (log A-log B).
    e. 10 (log B-log A).

24. Regarding audible sound levels,
    a. 0 dB means no sound.
    b. 0 dB is the threshold of hearing.
    c. normal office sounds should be 70 dB.
    d. the threshold of hearing is 70 dB.
    e. the threshold of pain is 70 dB.

25. Ultrasound amplitude
    a. increases with increasing frequency.
    b. is a measure of particle displacement.
    c. is measured in MHz/cm^2.
    d. is the same as ultrasonic power.
    e. is a measure of ultrasound velocity.

26. Acoustic impedance increases with increasing
    a. frequency.
    b. wavelength.
    c. mass.
    d. mass density.
    e. optical density.

27. When an ultrasound beam is attenuated by soft tissue,
    a. a 3 dB loss is equivalent to a 50% reduction.
    b. a 6 dB loss is equivalent to a 100% reduction.
    c. a 100 dB loss is equivalent to a 100% reduction.
    d. the average rate is 1 dB/cm/MHz.
    e. the average rate is 10 dB/cm/MHz.

28. Which of the following statements is true regarding ultrasound attenuation in matter?
    a. A good rule of thumb is 1 half-value layer (HVL)/mm/MHz.
    b. The principal attenuating effects are recombinant effects.
    c. Acoustic impedance is the product of mass density and velocity.
    d. Acoustic impedance is the product of mass density and frequency.
    e. The unit of acoustic impedance is mW/cm^2.

29. Which of the following is equivalent to doubling the signal intensity?

    a. 1 dB
    b. 3 dB
    c. 5 dB
    d. 10 dB
    e. 20 dB

30. If a reflected wave has to be amplified by a factor of 20 in order to have the same intensity as the transmitted wave, it will be amplified

    a. 3 dB.
    b. 10 dB.
    c. 13 dB.
    d. 20 dB.
    e. 23 dB.

31. The decibel is defined as

    a. $1/10 \log (I_r/I_t)$.
    b. $10 \log (I_r/I_t)$.
    c. $1/10 \log (I_t/I_r)$.
    d. $10 \log (I_t/I_r)$.
    e. $10 \log (I_t - I_r)$.

32. The threshold for pain by audible sound is approximately

    a. 50 dB.
    b. 70 dB.
    c. 90 dB.
    d. 110 dB.
    e. 130 dB.

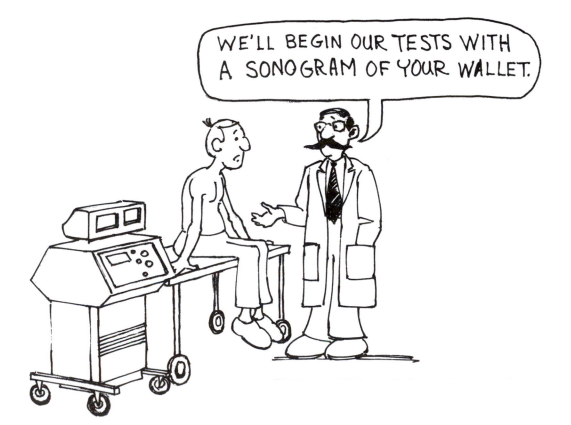

The Ultrasound Beam

- There are two kinds of diagnostic ultrasound beams—**continuous-wave (CW)** and **pulse echo (PE)**.

- Continuous-wave ultrasound is used for Doppler measurement of moving interfaces and blood.

- Pulse echo ultrasound is used for imaging.

- Wavelength (λ), frequency (f) and period (T) apply to both continuous and PE ultrasound.

ULTRASOUND BEAM SHAPE

- If emitted from a single-point transducer, ultrasound would appear as a **spherical wavefront**.

- When emitted from a large transducer, ultrasound appears as a **plane wavefront**.

- When emitted from multiple transducer elements in an array, ultrasound appears as a plane wavefront.

- The formation of the plane wavefront follows Huygens' principle.

- It is the plane wavefront that is used for Doppler ultrasound and PE imaging.

- **Side lobes** to the main beam often exist and can result in spurious images.

- Ultrasound beams consisting of plane waves have two distinct regions—the near field and the far field.

- The **near field**, or Fresnel zone, is closest to the transducer.

- The near field is highly collimated with great variation in intensity from wavefront to wavefront.

- Farther from the transducer face is the **far field**, or Fraunhofer zone.

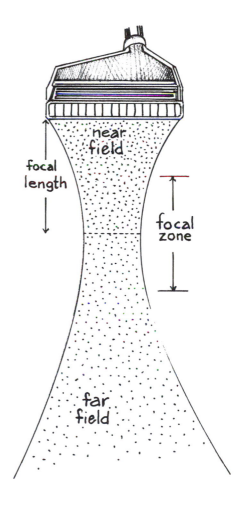

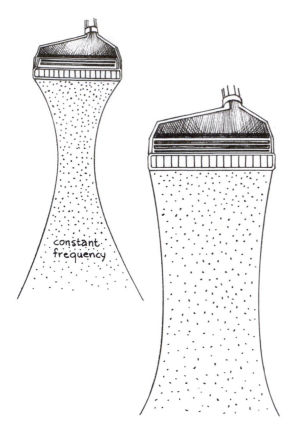

constant frequency

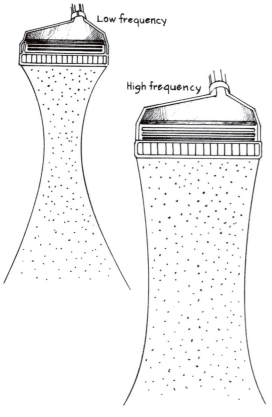

Low frequency

High frequency

- In the far field the ultrasound beam diverges and is more uniform in intensity from wavefront to wavefront.

- At the near field/far field transition, there is a modest reduction in the size of the cross section of the beam.

- Best imaging is obtained at the near field/far field transition.

- Best spatial resolution is obtained at the near field/far field transition.

- The near field/far field transition is sometimes called the **focal zone** or region.

- The diameter of the near field is approximately equal to the diameter of the transducer or transducer array.

- The length of the near field is a function of the size of the transducer, the frequency of ultrasound, and the velocity of ultrasound in that tissue.

- The far field is usually described by the angle of divergence, which, in turn, is a function of ultrasound frequency and the diameter of the transducer.

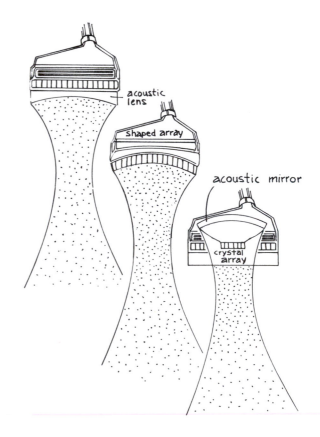

acoustic lens

Shaped array

acoustic mirror

crystal array

- In general, as transducer diameter is increased with constant frequency, the near field is lengthened and the far field diverges less.

- In general, as the ultrasound frequency is increased with a fixed-diameter transducer, the near field is lengthened and the far field diverges less.

- The ultrasound beam can be focused for better lateral resolution in the focal zone.

- Focusing is accomplished by acoustic lenses or a concave crystal shape.

- Focusing increases beam intensity in the focal zone.

PULSE ECHO ULTRASOUND

- A pulse of ultrasound usually contains three to five cycles.

- The **pulse repetition frequency (PRF)** is the number of pulses emitted per second. PRF is expressed in hertz (Hz).

- Increasing the PRF results in less time between pulses to receive echoes and therefore limits imaging depth.

- The time required from the beginning of one pulse, to the beginning of the next is the **pulse repetition period (PRP)**. PRP is expressed in milliseconds.

- The PRP and PRF are reciprocally related.

- The time during which the ultrasound pulse is actually emitted is the **pulse duration (PD)**. PD is expressed in microseconds.

- Pulse duration is equal to the product of the ultrasound period times the number of cycles in a pulse.

- The fraction of time the ultrasound pulse is actually being emitted during one PRP is called the **duty factor (DF)**.

- The duty factor is equal to the pulse duration divided by the pulse repetition period.

- The duty factor also equals the temporal average divided by the temporal peak.

- Duty factor has no units; it is a dimensionless number.

$$PRP = \frac{1}{PRF}$$

$$PRP_{max} = \frac{2 \times depth_{max}}{velocity}$$

$$PRF_{max} = \frac{velocity}{2 \times depth_{max}}$$

$$DF = \frac{PD\ (\mu s)}{PRP\ (ms) \times 1000}$$

$$DF = \frac{PD\ (\mu s) \times PRF\ (kHz)}{1000}$$

$$DF = TA/TP$$

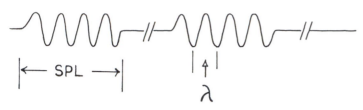

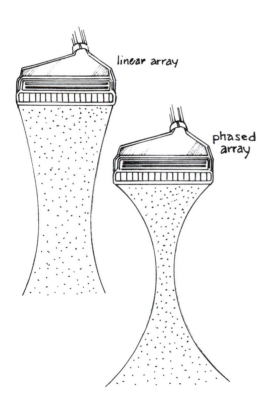

- Continuous-wave ultrasound has a duty factor equal to 1.

- Pulse echo ultrasound normally has a duty factor of <0.01.

- **Spatial pulse length** (SPL) is the length or space over which an ultrasound pulse occurs. SPL is expressed in millimeters.

- Spatial pulse length is the product of ultrasound wavelength multiplied by the number of cycles in a pulse.

- Spatial pulse length is very important for image resolution.

- The shorter the SPL, the better will be axial spatial resolution.

ULTRASOUND RESOLUTION

- Medical images exhibit several types of resolution.

- **Spatial resolution** is the ability to image small, high-contrast objects.

- Of all medical imaging, mammography has the best spatial resolution.

- **Contrast resolution** is the ability to distinguish one similar tissue from another.

- Of all medical imaging, magnetic resonance imaging (MRI) has the best contrast resolution.

- **Temporal resolution** is the ability to measure and quantitate motion.

- Fluoroscopy and real-time ultrasound have good temporal resolution.

- **Energy resolution** is the ability to measure and quantitate energy, as in gamma spectroscopy.

- Gamma cameras used in nuclear medicine have the best energy resolution.

- Diagnostic ultrasound has fair spatial, contrast, and temporal resolution.

- Energy resolution does not apply to diagnostic ultrasound.

- There are two important measures of spatial resolution in diagnostic ultrasound—axial resolution and lateral resolution.

- **Axial resolution** is the ability to image closely spaced interfaces along the axis of the ultrasound beam. Expressed in millimeters.

- Axial resolution is sometimes called range resolution, depth resolution, or longitudinal resolution.

- Axial resolution depends on three interrelated characteristics—SPL, ultrasound frequency, and damping.

- Spatial pulse length is equal to ultrasound wavelength times the number of cycles in a pulse.

- Short SPL results in better axial resolution.

- Higher ultrasound frequency results in a lengthened near field and a more collimated far field but less tissue penetration.

- Above approximately 10 MHz, penetration is too shallow for imaging.

- High ultrasound frequency results in better axial resolution at any depth and better lateral resolution in the far field.

- Below approximately 2 MHz, axial resolution is too poor for imaging.

- **Damping** refers to how quickly a pulse of ultrasound can be initiated and extinguished.

- Ultrasound with no damping will continue to oscillate for some time after the pulse is finished—this is called **ringdown**.

- Ultrasound that is highly damped will have little ringdown.

- The best single measure of axial resolution is the SPL.

- The best possible axial resolution is one-half the SPL.

- **Lateral resolution** is the ability to image closely spaced objects perpendicular to the axis of the ultrasound beam.

- Lateral resolution is sometimes called azimuthal resolution or transverse resolution.

- Lateral resolution is usually worse than axial resolution.

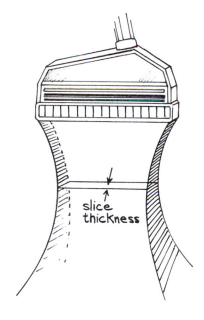

- Lateral resolution is determined by transducer size and beam width and somewhat by frequency.

- The smaller the transducer or transducer element, the better the lateral resolution.

- Lateral resolution is approximately equal to the effective ultrasound beam width.

- Lateral resolution is best at the depth of focus for a given transducer.

- Lateral resolution in the transverse plane parallel to an array can be improved by phased-array focusing.

- Lateral resolution in the transverse plane perpendicular to the array—or slice thickness—can be improved by focusing with an acoustic lens for each element.

- Lateral resolution in the transverse plane perpendicular to the array—or slice thickness—can be improved by using a curved piezoelectric crystal.

- With higher frequency, the ultrasound beam does not diverge so much in the far field; therefore, as compared with low frequency, lateral resolution is improved.

- Lateral resolution and slice thickness cannot be expressed precisely because the ultrasound beam does not have clearly defined edges.

$$PD = \#\,cycles \times T$$

$$SPL = \#\,cycles \times \lambda$$

$$axial\ resolution = \frac{SPL}{2}$$

Chapter 4 Review Questions

1. A 2.25 MHz three-cycle pulse of ultrasound is emitted at a pulse repetition frequency (PRF) of 500 pulses per second. What is the approximate pulse duration (PD)?

   a. 0.3 μs   d. 1.3 μs
   b. 0.4 μs   e. 2.0 μs
   c. 0.9 μs

2. Which equation is used to compute the degree of refraction?

   a. $Z = \rho v$ b. $v = \lambda f$ c. $dB = 10 \log \frac{I_t}{I_o}$

   d. $\dfrac{\sin_i}{\sin_r} = \dfrac{v_i}{v_r}$ e. $\left(\dfrac{Z_2 - Z_1}{Z_2 + Z_1}\right)^2$

3. **Best lateral resolution is obtained with**
    a. highest frequency and smallest transducer.
    b. highest frequency and largest transducer.
    c. lowest frequency and smallest transducer.
    d. lowest frequency and largest transducer.
    e. varies with tissue type.

4. **Axial resolution can be improved**
    1. by increasing frequency.
    2. with a lower Q value transducer.
    3. by reducing pulse length (PL).
    4. by using higher pulse repetition frequency (PRF).

    a. Only 1, 2, and 3 are correct.
    b. Only 1 and 3 are correct.
    c. Only 2 and 4 are correct.
    d. Only 4 is correct.
    e. All are correct.

5. **What is the approximate depth of the near field for a 10 mm diameter transducer operating at 2.25 MHz?**
    a. 20 mm   d. 120 mm
    b. 40 mm   e. 160 mm
    c. 80 mm

6. **Lateral resolution can be improved by**
    1. increasing frequency.
    2. adding an acoustic lens.
    3. reducing pulse repetition frequency (PRF).
    4. reducing transducer size.

    a. Only 1, 2, and 3 are correct.
    b. Only 1 and 3 are correct.
    c. Only 2 and 4 are correct.
    d. Only 4 is correct.
    e. All are correct.

7. **Temporal average intensity (TA) is equal to**
    a. pulse average intensity (PA) times duty factor (DF).
    b. pulse average intensity (PA) times spatial pulse length (SPL).
    c. spatial pulse length (SPL) times duty factor (DF).
    d. spatial pulse length (SPL) times frequency.
    e. spatial pulse length (SPL) times pulse repetition frequency (PRF).

8. **Which of the following has least value for pulse echo (PE) ultrasound?**
    a. SATA
    b. SPPA
    c. SATP
    d. SPTP
    e. SPTA

9. **Which of the following describes the frequency bandwidth of ultrasound?**
    a. impedance
    b. Q value
    c. Doppler
    d. Huygens' principle
    e. pulse duration (PD)

10. **What is the fraction of time that ultrasound is emitted?**
    a. Q value
    b. duty factor (DF)
    c. pulse duration (PD)
    d. spatial pulse length (SPL)
    e. pulse repetition frequency (PRF)

11. **When the number of cycles in a pulse is increased,**
    1. axial resolution is increased.
    2. lateral resolution is increased.
    3. attenuation increases.
    4. spatial pulse length (SPL) is increased.

    a. Only 1, 2, and 3 are correct.
    b. Only 1 and 3 are correct.
    c. Only 2 and 4 are correct.
    d. Only 4 is correct.
    e. All are correct.

12. **Which of the following describes far-field divergence?**
    a. $v = f\lambda$
    b. $v_t \sin_i = v_i \sin_t$
    c. $\sin_i = 1.22\ \lambda/d$
    d. $Z_i \sin_i = Z_t \sin_t$
    e. $d = \frac{1}{2} vt$

13. **Spatial pulse length (SPL)**
    1. affects depth of image.
    2. decreases with increasing frequency.
    3. improves lateral resolution.
    4. improves axial resolution.

    a. Only 1, 2, and 3 are correct.
    b. Only 1 and 3 are correct.
    c. Only 2 and 4 are correct.
    d. Only 4 is correct.
    e. All are correct.

14. **Axial resolution**
    1. improves with increasing intensity.
    2. is best at the focal length.
    3. improves with reduced transducer size.
    4. depends on wavelength.

    a. Only 1, 2, and 3 are correct.
    b. Only 1 and 3 are correct.
    c. Only 2 and 4 are correct.
    d. Only 4 is correct.
    e. All are correct.

15. **An ultrasound beam diverges**
    a. in the Fresnel zone.
    b. in the Fraunhofer zone.
    c. more with reduced transducer size.
    d. with increasing spatial pulse length (SPL).
    e. with increasing pulse repetition frequency (PRF).

16. **By reducing the spatial pulse length (SPL), one can improve**
    a. axial resolution.
    b. lateral resolution.
    c. temporal resolution.
    d. depth of field.
    e. pulse repetition frequency (PRF).

17. **The period of an ultrasound beam is best represented by**
    1. the inverse duty cycle.
    2. the inverse of frequency.
    3. the time between pulses.
    4. the time of one wavelength.

    a. Only 1, 2, and 3 are correct.
    b. Only 1 and 3 are correct.
    c. Only 2 and 4 are correct.
    d. Only 4 is correct.
    e. All are correct.

18. **Increasing the pulse repetition frequency (PRF) will**
    a. reduce the depth of image.
    b. increase the depth of image.
    c. reduce axial resolution.
    d. increase axial resolution.
    e. shorten examination time.

19. **Axial resolution is improved with**
    a. smaller-diameter crystal.
    b. larger-diameter crystal.
    c. lower frequency.
    d. higher frequency.
    e. thinner matching layer.

20. **Which term describes the fraction of time during pulse echo (PE) imaging that ultrasound is actually emitted?**
    a. activation time
    b. bandwidth
    c. duty cycle
    d. pulse length
    e. pulse repetition rate (PRR)

21. **The center frequency of an ultrasound pulse divided by its bandwidth is called**
    1. modulation factor.
    2. quality factor (QF).
    3. homogeneity factor.
    4. Q value.

    a. Only 1, 2, and 3 are correct.
    b. Only 1 and 3 are correct.
    c. Only 2 and 4 are correct.
    d. Only 4 is correct.
    e. All are correct.

22. Ultrasound emitted from the edges of a transducer element and not included in the primary beam is a/an
    a. artifact pulse.
    b. phantom pulse.
    c. side lobe.
    d. suppressed pulse.
    e. wide lobe.

23. What is the product of the number of cycles in a pulse and the pulse period called?
    a. pulse duration (PD)
    b. pulse repetition frequency (PRF)
    c. pulse frequency
    d. pulse repetition period (PRP)
    e. pulse homogeneity

24. Far-field dispersion can be reduced by using
    1. a real-time transducer.
    2. a larger transducer.
    3. shorter pulse repetition frequency (PRF).
    4. higher frequency.

    a. Only 1, 2, and 3 are correct.
    b. Only 1 and 3 are correct.
    c. Only 2 and 4 are correct.
    d. Only 4 is correct.
    e. All are correct.

25. PRF = pulse repetition frequency and SPL = spatial pulse length. Which of the following defines axial resolution?
    a. $2 \times SPL$
    b. $SPL/2$
    c. $2 \times PRF$
    d. $PRF/2$
    e. SPL/PRF

26. Which of the following measurably influences axial resolution?
    1. frequency
    2. damping
    3. spatial pulse length (SPL)
    4. crystal size

    a. Only 1, 2, and 3 are correct.
    b. Only 1 and 3 are correct.
    c. Only 2 and 4 are correct.
    d. Only 4 is correct.
    e. All are correct.

27. If f is center frequency and Δf the frequency bandwidth, what is $f/\Delta f$?
    a. frequency spread
    b. frequency homogeneity
    c. Q value
    d. R value
    e. S value

28. An increase in ultrasound frequency will result in

    1. shorter wavelength.
    2. deeper penetration.
    3. better axial resolution.
    4. better lateral resolution.

    a. Only 1, 2, and 3 are correct.
    b. Only 1 and 3 are correct.
    c. Only 2 and 4 are correct.
    d. Only 4 is correct.
    e. All are correct.

29. Which equation is used to compute attenuation?

    a. $Z = \rho v$

    b. $v = \lambda f$

    c. $dB = 10 \log \dfrac{I_t}{I_o}$

    d. $\dfrac{\sin_i}{\sin_r} = \dfrac{v_i}{v_r}$

    e. $\left(\dfrac{Z_2 - Z_1}{Z_2 + Z_1} \right)^2$

30. A 2.25 MHz three-cycle pulse of ultrasound is emitted at a pulse repetition frequency (PRF) of 500 pulses per second. What is the approximate spatial pulse length (SPL) in soft tissue?

    a. 1 mm
    b. 2 mm
    c. 3 mm
    d. 4 mm
    e. 5 mm

31. Ultrasound frequency is inversely proportional to

    1. velocity.
    2. period.
    3. intensity.
    4. wavelength.

    a. Only 1, 2, and 3 are correct.
    b. Only 1 and 3 are correct.
    c. Only 2 and 4 are correct.
    d. Only 4 is correct.
    e. All are correct.

32. Axial resolution is also called

    1. depth resolution.
    2. longitudinal resolution.
    3. range resolution.
    4. azimuthal resolution.

    a. Only 1, 2, and 3 are correct.
    b. Only 1 and 3 are correct.
    c. Only 2 and 4 are correct.
    d. Only 4 is correct.
    e. All are correct.

33. The beam uniformity ratio is defined as
    a. SA/SP.
    b. SP/SA.
    c. TA/TP.
    d. TP/TA.
    e. SA/TA.

34. Pulse echo (PE) imaging usually employs a duty cycle of what percent?
    a. <1
    b. 1 to 5
    c. 5 to 10
    d. 10 to 25
    e. 100

35. Reducing spatial pulse length (SPL) results in
    a. deeper penetration.
    b. higher Q value.
    c. lower intensity.
    d. reduced reflectivity.
    e. improved axial resolution.

36. A transducer with high Q value will have a bandwidth described as
    1. high.
    2. low.
    3. wide.
    4. narrow.

    a. Only 1, 2, and 3 are correct.
    b. Only 1 and 3 are correct.
    c. Only 2 and 4 are correct.
    d. Only 4 is correct.
    e. All are correct.

37. Axial resolution is improved by
    a. increasing intensity.
    b. using a smaller transducer.
    c. reducing the pulse repetition frequency (PRF).
    d. reducing the spatial pulse length (SPL).
    e. increasing the period.

38. Lateral resolution is also known as
    1. azimuthal resolution.
    2. angular resolution.
    3. transverse resolution.
    4. range resolution.

    a. Only 1, 2, and 3 are correct.
    b. Only 1 and 3 are correct.
    c. Only 2 and 4 are correct.
    d. Only 4 is correct.
    e. All are correct.

39. During pulse echo (PE) imaging, approximately what percent of the time can the transducer receive echoes?

    a. <1
    b. 1 to 5
    c. 10 to 25
    d. 99.9
    e. 100

40. Which of the following changes with depth into tissue?

    1. spatial pulse length (SPL)
    2. frequency
    3. axial resolution
    4. lateral resolution

    a. Only 1, 2, and 3 are correct.
    b. Only 1 and 3 are correct.
    c. Only 2 and 4 are correct.
    d. Only 4 is correct.
    e. All are correct.

41. What happens when frequency is increased?

    1. reduced penetration
    2. shorter spatial pulse length (SPL)
    3. better axial resolution
    4. better lateral resolution

    a. Only 1, 2, and 3 are correct.
    b. Only 1 and 3 are correct.
    c. Only 2 and 4 are correct.
    d. Only 4 is correct.
    e. All are correct.

42. Q value

    a. has units of MHz.
    b. has units of mW/cm^2.
    c. has units of rayl.
    d. has units of dB.
    e. is unitless.

43. During pulse echo (PE) imaging, the fraction of time that the transducer actually emits ultrasound is the

    a. spatial pulse length (SPL).
    b. period.
    c. pulse repetition frequency (PRF).
    d. Q value.
    e. duty factor (DF).

44. **The length of the near field can be increased by increasing**

    1. spatial pulse length (SPL).
    2. frequency.
    3. pulse repetition frequency (PRF).
    4. transducer diameter.

    a. Only 1, 2, and 3 are correct.
    b. Only 1 and 3 are correct.
    c. Only 2 and 4 are correct.
    d. Only 4 is correct.
    e. All are correct.

45. **The product of pulse duration (PD) and pulse repetition frequency (PRF) is**

    a. duty factor (DF).
    b. Q value.
    c. impedance.
    d. intensity.
    e. power.

46. **Which of the following is an example of an acoustic window?**

    a. bladder
    b. blood
    c. bone
    d. muscle/fat interface
    e. rib/lung interface

47. **Spatial pulse length (SPL) is the product of**

    a. pulse repetition frequency (PRF) and frequency.
    b. pulse repetition frequency (PRF) and wavelength.
    c. duty cycle and wavelength.
    d. wavelength and cycles per pulse.
    e. duty cycle and cycles per pulse.

48. **In pulse echo (PE) ultrasound, the range of frequencies in a pulse is the**

    a. bandwidth.
    b. duty cycle.
    c. Q value.
    d. rms value.
    e. spatial frequency.

49. **Reducing pulse duration (PD) will improve**

    a. axial resolution.
    b. bandwidth.
    c. duty cycle.
    d. lateral resolution.
    e. Q value.

50. **For an unfocused transducer, the near-field length depends on**

    a. backing material and wavelength.
    b. crystal diameter and frequency.
    c. crystal thickness and wavelength.
    d. matching layer and crystal diameter.
    e. matching layer and frequency.

51. What is the percent duty factor (DF) for a pulse echo (PE) beam having a 3 μs pulse duration (PD) and a 900 μs pulse repetition period (PRP)?

    a. 0.1
    b. 0.3
    c. 1
    d. 3
    e. 10

52. Frequency of operation significantly influences

    1. compressibility.
    2. tissue attenuation.
    3. ultrasound velocity.
    4. axial resolution.

    a. Only 1, 2, and 3 are correct.
    b. Only 1 and 3 are correct.
    c. Only 2 and 4 are correct.
    d. Only 4 is correct.
    e. All are correct.

53. Which of the following is correct regarding lateral resolution?

    1. usually better than axial resolution
    2. improves at higher frequency
    3. approximately equal throughout imaging depth
    4. approximately equal to beam diameter

    a. Only 1, 2, and 3 are correct.
    b. Only 1 and 3 are correct.
    c. Only 2 and 4 are correct.
    d. Only 4 is correct.
    e. All are correct.

54. When the pulse repetition period (PRP) is increased,

    a. axial resolution is improved.
    b. depth of image is lengthened.
    c. duty factor (DF) is increased.
    d. lateral resolution is improved.
    e. Q value is reduced.

55. The intensity of a focused ultrasound beam is highest

    a. at the transducer/skin interface.
    b. at the skin.
    c. in the near zone.
    d. at the focal zone.
    e. in the far zone.

56. Transmitted ultrasound pulses containing a narrow bandwidth will have

    a. better lateral resolution.
    b. less penetration.
    c. a low Q value.
    d. poorer axial resolution.
    e. reduced duty factor (DF).

57. A 5 μs pulse is emitted every 500 μs. What is the pulse repetition period (PRP)?

    a. 0.5 ms
    b. 5.0 ms
    c. 500 pulses/ms
    d. 500 pulses/s
    e. 2000 pulses/s

58. The intensity of ultrasound is most uniform

    a. in the piezoelectric crystal.
    b. in the superficial skin.
    c. in the near field.
    d. at the near field–far field transition.
    e. in the far field.

59. Five cycles of 1 MHz ultrasound are emitted per pulse with a pulse repetition rate (PRR) of 1000 pulses per second. What is the duty factor (DF)?

    a. 0.001
    b. 0.005
    c. 0.01
    d. 0.05
    e. 0.1

60. A 4.5 MHz ultrasound beam will have a period of approximately

    a. 0.02 μs.
    b. 0.1 μs.
    c. 0.2 μs.
    d. 0.4 μs.
    e. 0.5 μs.

61. When radiation is emitted isotropically, it is emitted

    a. as a highly collimated beam.
    b. as a broadly scattered beam.
    c. with equal intensity in all directions.
    d. with equal velocity in all directions.
    e. with equal phase and frequency.

62. Which of the following designations will have the highest value for pulse echo (PE) ultrasound?

    a. SATA
    b. SPTA
    c. SATP
    d. SPTP
    e. SPPA

63. Which of the following will increase as the frequency of ultrasound increases?

    a. intensity
    b. velocity
    c. penetration in tissue
    d. wavelength
    e. axial resolution

64. **The resolution of a diagnostic ultrasound imager is**
    1. usually best perpendicular to the axis of the beam.
    2. dependent on the spatial pulse length (SPL).
    3. usually best in the far field.
    4. dependent on the frequency of operation.

    a. Only 1, 2, and 3 are correct.
    b. Only 1 and 3 are correct.
    c. Only 2 and 4 are correct.
    d. Only 4 is correct.
    e. All are correct.

65. **Best spatial resolution is obtained**
    a. in the superficial skin.
    b. in the near field.
    c. at the near field–far field transition.
    d. in the far field.
    e. beyond the far field.

66. **The Fraunhofer zone is the**
    a. image plane.
    b. image focus plane.
    c. image focal zone.
    d. near field.
    e. far field.

67. **Best axial resolution is obtained with**
    a. highest frequency and shortest spatial pulse length (SPL).
    b. highest frequency and longest spatial pulse length (SPL).
    c. lowest frequency and shortest spatial pulse length (SPL).
    d. lowest frequency and longest spatial pulse length (SPL).
    e. varies with tissue type.

68. **A 2.25 MHz three-cycle pulse of ultrasound is emitted at a pulse repetition frequency (PRF) of 500 pulses per second. What is the approximate duty factor (DF)?**
    a. 0.09
    b. 0.005
    c. 0.009
    d. 0.0005
    e. 0.0009

69. **Which of the following statements best characterizes the ultrasound beam?**
    a. If the crystal diameter is large, a plane wavefront is formed.
    b. Best resolution is obtained in the far field.
    c. As frequency is increased, the near field is lengthened.
    d. As the transducer diameter is increased, the near field shrinks.
    e. The Q value is the relative time the beam exists.

70. **The lateral ultrasound resolution is**
    a. also called azimuthal resolution.
    b. also called range resolution.
    c. better in the near field.
    d. better with lower frequency.
    e. better than axial resolution.

71. Five cycles of 2 MHz ultrasound are emitted per pulse. What is the approximate pulse duration (PD)?

    a. 0.5 μs
    b. 1.0 μs
    c. 2.5 μs
    d. 5.0 μs
    e. 7.5 μs

72. The Q value is principally a function of

    a. resonant frequency and acoustic impedance (Z).
    b. resonant frequency and bandwidth.
    c. bandwidth and pulse duration (PD).
    d. bandwidth and acoustic impedance (Z).
    e. acoustic impedance (Z) and bandwidth.

73. Which of the following primarily depends on the pulse duration (PD)?

    a. axial resolution
    b. lateral resolution
    c. contrast resolution
    d. reflectivity
    e. Q value

74. Which of the following will best produce a long Fresnel zone?

    a. reduce crystal diameter
    b. increase crystal diameter
    c. reduce damping
    d. increase damping
    e. increase the thickness of matching layer

The Ultrasound Imager

- A **transducer** is any device that converts energy from one form to another.

- An ultrasound transducer converts electrical energy to mechanical energy and vice versa.

- The emitting and receiving element of an ultrasound transducer is a **piezoelectric crystal**.

- The emitted ultrasound beam obeys **Huygens' principle**—the resultant wavefront is the combination of individual wavelets emitted from different regions of the transducer face or from multiple transducer elements.

RESONANCE

- A piezoelectric crystal will alternately expand and contract along its short axis when the polarity of an electrical signal across the crystal is reversed.

- An ultrasound transducer converts an electrical signal into mechanical energy, which is the ultrasound beam.

- Reflected ultrasound echoes are detected by the transducer, which converts this mechanical energy into an electrical signal.

- Piezoelectric crystals are made of various materials—quartz, lithium niobate, lithium sulfate, ceramic materials, lead zirconate titanate (PZT), barium titanate, and lead metaniobate.

- Lead zirconate titanate is the material of choice for most transducer elements because of its superior efficiency, higher sensitivity, availability, and low cost.

- Lead zirconate titanate is a ceramic that is easily shaped for focusing.

- The critical dimension of a piezoelectric crystal is its thickness.

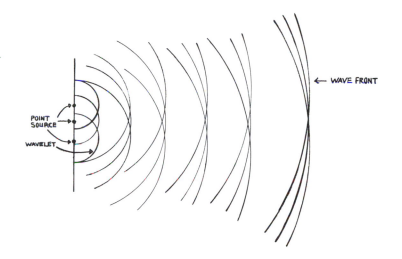

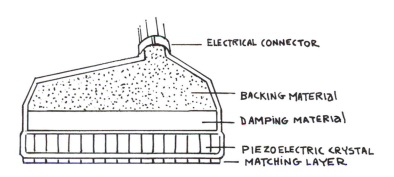

$$d = \tfrac{1}{2}\, v t$$

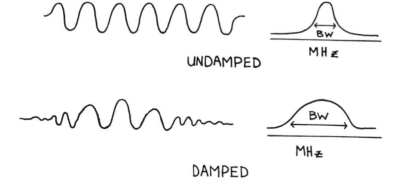

UNDAMPED

DAMPED

- For maximum efficiency, the thickness of a piezoelectric crystal should be one-half the wavelength of the ultrasound produced by the crystal.

- When the thickness of the piezoelectric crystal is one-half wavelength, complete constructive interference—**resonance**—is obtained.

- Thinner piezoelectric crystals have higher-resonance frequencies.

- The diameter of the crystal has no effect on frequency.

- Immediately behind the piezoelectric crystal is **damping material**. Epoxy resin and tungsten powder serve as damping material, which reduces the ringdown of an emitted ultrasound pulse.

- Damping increases bandwidth.

- The use of damping material in a PE transducer reduces the spatial pulse length (SPL) and the pulse duration (PD) and improves axial resolution.

- Continuous-wave (CW) ultrasound is not damped; rather, the crystal is backed with air.

- Sandwiched between the piezoelectric crystal and the patient's skin is a **matching layer** and **acoustic coupling**.

- A matching layer is fashioned to be one-quarter wavelength and of intermediate acoustic impedance between that of the piezoelectric crystal and soft tissue.

- Multiple matching layers are often used.

- Acoustic coupling between the transducer and the patient's skin consists of copious amounts of gel or mineral oil.

- If air is trapped between transducer and skin, essentially all ultrasound is reflected and none is available for imaging.

- The very low acoustic impedance of air results in very high reflectivity.

- Both the matching layer and the acoustic coupling permit more ultrasound energy to be transmitted into the patient and less reflected at the skin.

- The range of frequencies present in an ultrasound beam is termed the **bandwidth** of the beam.

- There is increased bandwidth with increased damping.

- The shorter the spatial pulse length, the broader the bandwidth.

- Continuous-wave (CW) ultrasound has a narrow bandwidth. A CW beam contains essentially one frequency.

- Pulse echo ultrasound has a wider bandwidth. Short SPL means fewer cycles per pulse, more frequencies, and wider bandwidth.

- The **Q value** describes the frequency homogeneity of the ultrasound beam.

- Q value is equal to the resonance frequency divided by the bandwidth.

- Generally, the narrower the bandwidth of an ultrasound beam, the higher will be the Q value.

- Transducers with low Q value have a short ringdown, resulting in short SPL; therefore they are better for imaging.

- Q value increases with increasing frequency.

- Q value is a number without units.

THE RANGE EQUATION

- Pulse echo (PE) imaging applies the range equation to determine distance to a tissue interface.

- The **range equation** states that the distance (*d*) to a tissue interface is equal to one-half the product of the velocity (*v*) of sound in that tissue and the time (*t*) between the emitted pulse and the echo.

- Ultrasound images are calibrated at the velocity of ultrasound in soft tissue—1540 m/s.

OPERATIONAL MODES

- There are three principal operational modes for PE ultrasound—amplitude mode (A-mode), brightness mode (B-mode) and motion mode (M-mode).

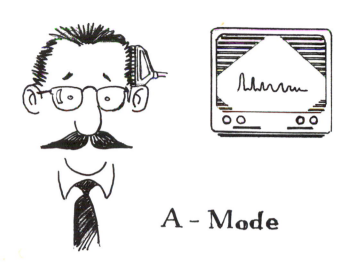

A - Mode

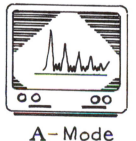

A-Mode

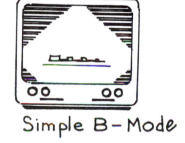

Simple B-Mode

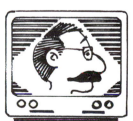

Compound B-Mode

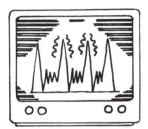

A – Mode

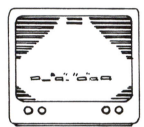

B – Mode

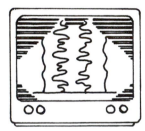

M – Mode

- Each of these three modes measures (1) an intensity of reflected echoes, (2) time required for reflection, and (3) direction from which the echo was reflected.

- For A-mode ultrasound, echoes appear on a cathode ray tube (CRT) as a series of blips.

- For A-mode imaging, the distance between blips is proportional to the distance between interfaces.

- For A-mode imaging, the height of each blip is proportional to the intensity of each echo.

- For A-mode imaging, distal reflections produce smaller blips than proximal reflections.

- A-mode imaging is used principally to measure the depth of interfaces and their separation accurately.

- A-mode ultrasound equipment is relatively inexpensive.

- For B-mode imaging, the intensity of the echo is represented by a bright dot on the CRT.

- B-mode imaging can be done with a single transducer element, which is properly moved by the ultrasonographer during the examination.

- Today all B-mode imaging is performed with a multielement transducer array—the realtime imager.

- Depending upon transducer design, B-mode images will be formatted as rectangular or sector views.

- A scan converter is a special type of CRT, which stores B-mode signals as they are received and displays them on the CRT as a composite image.

- M-mode imaging is used to examine moving interfaces, such as cardiac wall motion.

- M-mode imaging has been replaced by dedicated echocardiographic imagers incorporating B-mode and Doppler ultrasound.

- M-mode imaging renders the intensity of an A-mode echo along a time axis rather than a space axis.

- The information contained in M-mode ultrasound appears as a strip-chart recorder not unlike an electrocardiogram (ECG) or electroencephalogram (EEG).

REALTIME IMAGERS

- Realtime imaging is possible because of the development of the digital scan converter and the microprocessor.

- Realtime imaging is to diagnostic ultrasound as fluoroscopy is to x ray imaging—both are called **dynamic imaging**.

- The following are distinct advantages to realtime imaging: (1) quick image acquisition, (2) ease of image acquisition, (3) continuous image appearance with changing transducer position, (4) moving internal structures are imaged, and (5) portable imaging is possible.

- Realtime imaging is possible with mechanical movement of a single transducer or acoustic mirror or with electronic excitement of an array of transducer elements.

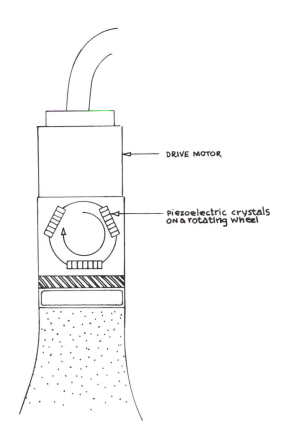

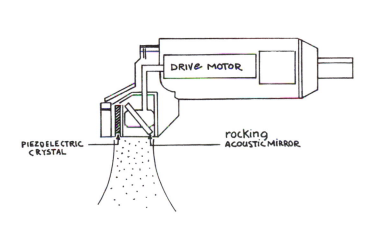

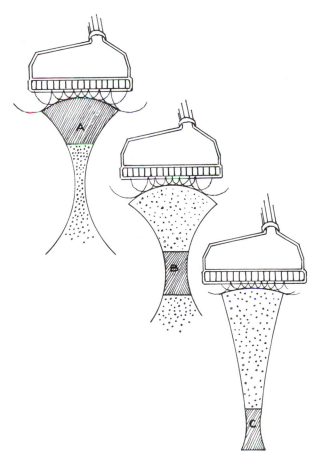

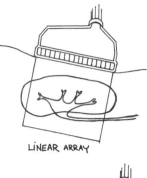

LINEAR ARRAY

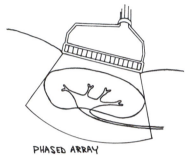

PHASED ARRAY

- There are several types of realtime imagers—mechanical, annular array, linear array, curvilinear array, and phased array.

- Mechanical realtime imagers have been designed around rotating, translating, and rocking transducers and a rocking acoustic mirror.

- Single-element beam focusing is accomplished with a concave transducer or a convex lens.

- Annular arrays can also be phased in order to obtain dynamic focusing at various depths.

- Linear arrays typically incorporate up to 600 transducer elements.

- Phased arrays typically incorporate up to 256 transducer elements.

- **Line density (LD)** is the number of lines in an image.

- Higher LD results in better image quality.

- Line density for a rectangular display is the number of lines divided by the display width.

- Line density for a sector display is the number of lines divided by the display angle.

- The time required to obtain a complete image is determined by the line density and depth of image.

- The frequency with which an image is refreshed during realtime imaging is called the **frame rate (FR)**.

- Frame rate affects image flicker.

- The integration time of the eye is approximately 200 ms, which corresponds to an FR of five frames per second.

$$time = 13\mu s \times LD \times depth$$

$$PRF = FR \times LD$$

$$depth\,(cm) = \frac{77,000}{FR \times LD}$$

$$depth\,(cm) = \frac{77,000}{PRF}$$

- Flicker is visible up to about 20 frames per second.

- Cardiac imaging requires at least 30 frames per second.

- The **pulse repetition frequency (PRF)** determines the rate at which transducer elements are energized.

- The PRF is the product of FR and LD.

- The PRF is limited by the maximum depth of the image because of the transit time in tissue, 6.5 μs/cm.

- In order to image deep tissues, a lower PRF is required.

- Maximum image depth is also determined by the velocity of sound in tissue (1540 m/s), or actually one-half that value (77,000 cm/s) because of the round trip.

- **Rectangular images** are produced by linear-array realtime transducers, either sequentially or segmentally activated.

- Linear array is a misnomer, since these arrays are fabricated straight or curved.

- **Sector scans** are produced by phased-array or mechanical realtime transducers.

- **Sequential activation** occurs when one transducer element after another is individually energized during imaging.

- Simultaneous activation of groups of transducer elements is **segmental activation**.

- Segmental activation uses each transducer element several times in an image frame, resulting in increased signal-to-noise ratio.

- Phased-array transducer elements can be energized sequentially or segmentally.

- The term **phase** refers to a very slight difference in timing of ultrasound emission from one transducer element to the next.

- Phased-array multielement transducers produce ultrasound beams that can be steered and focused.

Q: Require a 15cm image depth at 30 frames/s. What will be the line density and PRF?

A: line density = $\frac{77,000}{30\ f/s \times 15\ cm}$ = 171 lines

PRF = $\frac{77,000}{15\ cm}$ = 5130 pulses/s

or PRF = 30 f/s × 171 lines = 5130 pulses/s

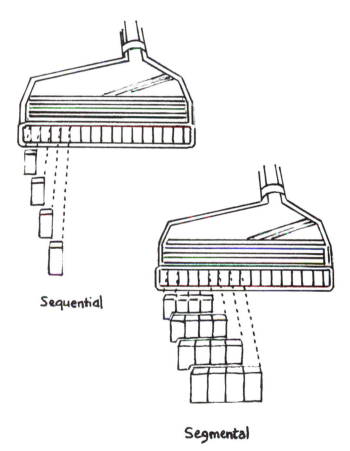

Sequential

Segmental

Suggested Transducer Selection

straight linear array	Curved linear array	Sector Scanner
breast carotid muscles penis testis	obstetrics	abdomen cardiology gynecology neonatal

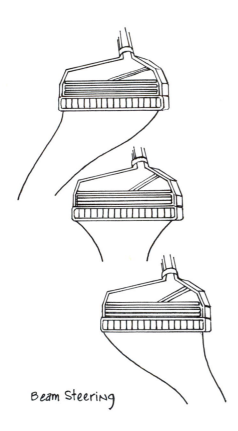

Beam Steering

Pulser:
- forms US pulse
- tells receiver to expect echo
- tells scan converter to expect echo
- controls pulse steering and focusing
- applies dynamic apodization

- Beam focusing in the scan plane is accomplished by the phased excitation of the transducer elements.

- Beam focusing of the width of the scan, slice thickness, is accomplished with an acoustic lens or shaped transducer elements.

- Dynamic focusing at multiple depths in possible.

- Ultrasound **side lobes** are produced perpendicular to the axis of the ultrasound beam.

- The presence of side lobes reduces image contrast resolution.

- **Apodization** reduces side lobe interference, resulting in improved contrast resolution and dynamic range.

- Apodization is accomplished electronically by varying pulse amplitude to the various transducer elements.

- **Grating lobes** are unwanted intensity lobes created by interference patterns of the multi-element array.

- Grating lobes can be reduced by reducing element size and increasing element number.

IMAGE PROCESSING AND DISPLAY

- The principal electronic components in an ultrasound imager are the **pulser, receiver, scan converter,** and **image display device.**

- In realtime imaging, each transducer element transmits a pulse of ultrasound into the patient and receives an echo some time later.

- The pulser applies an oscillating voltage to each transducer element at the rate of 1000 to 5000 pulses per second.

- The pulser determines the pulse repetition frequency (PRF)—1 to 5 kHz as in the previous statement.

- The amplitude of the voltage applied by the pulser to each transducer element determines the intensity of the emitted ultrasound beam.

- The pulser signals the receiver to be ready for an echo.

- Echoes vary over a wide intensity range. The deeper the reflecting tissue interface, the weaker will be the echo.

- The ultrasound receiver has an **amplification range** or **gain** of up to 120 decibels.

- The receiver performs the following functions: **amplification**, **compensation**, **compression**, **demodulation**, and **rejection**.

- Amplification range is also called **dynamic range**, but **gain** is usually used.

- The higher the gain of the amplifier, the better will be its sensitivity to weak echoes.

- **Time-gain compensation (TGC)** is an operator-controlled amplification of echoes.

- Time-gain compensation is manipulated to compensate for frequency, tissue-type attenuation, and depth of reflector.

- Reflections from deep interfaces are amplified more than those from shallow interfaces, so that image intensity is nearly uniform, resulting in equal brightness.

- Compression is the opposite of TGC.

- Compression reduces the amplitude of very large echoes; again, resulting in equal image brightness.

- Demodulation is performed on the ultrasound echo, converting it from an oscillating signal (AC) to a direct signal (DC).

- Demodulation involves rectification and filtering (smoothing).

- During the process of demodulation, the varying signal intensity of the ultrasound echo is smoothed by an electronic process called **enveloping**.

- Rejection is the suppression or elimination of very weak echoes below a given threshold.

- Rejection produces a less noisy-appearing image.

- Compression and rejection narrows the dynamic range of echoes to approximately 30 dB, that of the eye.

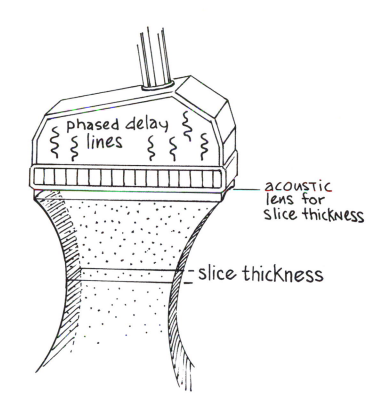

acoustic lens for slice thickness

slice thickness

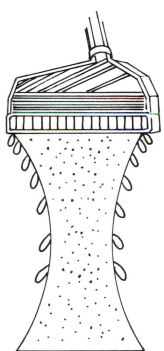

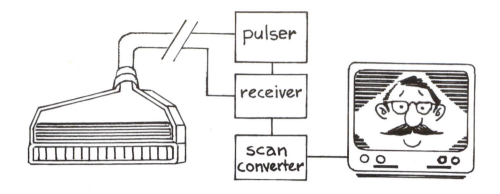

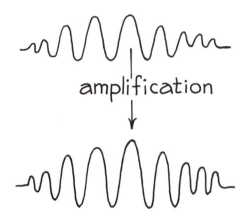

amplification

depth (time) ⟶

time gain compensation

- Video **scan converters** are available to handle either analog or digital signals.

- Only digital scan converters are currently used in diagnostic ultrasound.

- A scan converter is a special type of memory device incorporating a microprocessor.

- The scan converter is also a special type of video picture tube that stores signals in random-access memory (RAM), so that a full frame can be presented rather than sequential line tracings.

- Digital scan converters produce digital images formatted as a pixel matrix.

- Digital ultrasound imagers are becoming ever more common.

Receiver :
- amplifies
- compensates
- compresses
- demodulates
- rejects

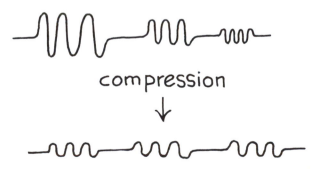

compression

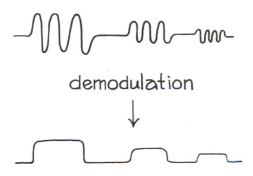

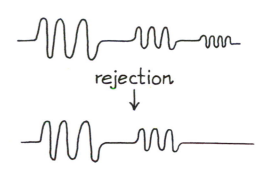

- A principal advantage to digital ultrasound is the ability to postprocess the image for improved contrast resolution.

- **Frame averaging** combines several images in order to reduce noise, thereby increasing signal-to-noise ratio (SNR) and improving image contrast.

- SNR is increased by the square root of the number of images averaged.

- The disadvantage of frame averaging is misregistration due to patient motion.

- Ultrasound images are normally displayed on a cathode ray tube (CRT).

- The display can be analog or the ever-increasing digital mode.

- Image matrix size and dynamic range are the principal characteristics of a digital image.

- The large matrix size (e.g., 512^2 vs. 256^2) improves spatial resolution.

- High dynamic range (e.g., 8 bit, 256 shades of gray vs. 4 bit, 16 shades of gray) improves contrast resolution.

- Color-flow Doppler requires higher dynamic range than gray scale in order to code the three primary colors in binary.

- Hard-copy film images are made with a Polaroid camera, laser camera, or color printer.

- Images are recorded to be viewed by others for comparison with earlier images and for teaching purposes.

# images combined	total signal	total noise	SNR
1	1	1	1
2	2	1.4	1.4
4	4	2	2
8	8	2.8	2.9
12	12	3.5	3.4

dynamic range	shades of gray
7 bit	128
8 bit	256
9 bit	512
10 bit	1024

- Windowing, leveling, and evaluation of a **region of interest (ROI)** are the principal post-processing features of image resolution.

- Linear area and circumference measurements are postprocessing analytical tools used to assign numerical values to anatomic structures; e.g., fetal head and abdomen measurement.

- Magnification, zoom, and pan are additional postprocessing features.

- Histogram analysis, mean, and standard deviation computation can be used to estimate tissue types within a region of interest (ROI).

Chapter 5 Review Questions

1. The Q value of an ultrasound transducer is a function of
   a. pulse duration (PD).
   b. frequency bandwidth.
   c. transmitted intensity.
   d. reflected intensity.
   e. duty factor (DF).

2. The matching layer of a transducer is designed to
   a. vary frequency of the beam.
   b. reduce refractivity.
   c. vary pulse duration (PD).
   d. reduce absorption.
   e. reduce reflectivity.

3. Removing the negative region of a pulse echo (PE) can be done by which signal processing technique?
   a. aliasing
   b. enveloping
   c. rectification
   d. windowing
   e. compression

4. Signal processing to reject weak echoes is done by
   a. enveloping.
   b. integration.
   c. thresholding.
   d. windowing.
   e. compression.

5. Which of the following is most often used as the piezoelectric crystal for realtime imaging?

   a. CsI   d. PZT
   b. BGO   e. quartz
   c. NaI

6. Which of the following is required for B mode but not A mode?

   a. pulse amplifier
   b. pulse attenuation
   c. scan converter
   d. time-gain control
   e. time-gain compensation (TGC)

7. A realtime image consists of 256 lines and the scanning depth is 6 cm. What is the approximate maximum frame rate (FR)?

   a. 10 frames per second
   b. 16 frames per second
   c. 20 frames per second
   d. 32 frames per second
   e. 50 frames per second

8. Which of the following can be used to focus an ultrasound beam?

   1. curved crystal   3. acoustic lens
   2. acoustic mirror   4. phased-element excitation

   a. Only 1, 2, and 3 are correct.
   b. Only 1 and 3 are correct.
   c. Only 2 and 4 are correct.
   d. Only 4 is correct.
   e. All are correct.

9. What is the approximate pixel size of a 256 $\times$ 256 matrix covering a 10 $\times$ 10 cm field of view?

   a. 0.1 $\times$ 0.1 mm
   b. 0.4 $\times$ 0.4 mm
   c. 0.8 $\times$ 0.8 mm
   d. 1.0 $\times$ 1.0 mm
   e. 1.2 $\times$ 1.2 mm

10. Conventional and digital television refresh images at what frame rate (FR)?

   a. 16 frames per second
   b. 30 frames per second
   c. 32 frames per second
   d. 48 frames per second
   e. 64 frames per second

11. Electronic focusing of a realtime ultrasound beam uses

   a. a curved crystal.
   b. time delay circuitry.
   c. acoustic lenses.
   d. variable pulse duration (PD).
   e. enveloping electronics.

12. Along the in-plane axis of a realtime ultrasound beam, lateral resolution is determined by
    1. beam width.
    2. image lines.
    3. matrix size.
    4. element size.

    a. Only 1, 2, and 3 are correct.
    b. Only 1 and 3 are correct.
    c. Only 2 and 4 are correct.
    d. Only 4 is correct.
    e. All are correct.

13. How does the ultrasonographer control the dynamic range of displayed echoes?
    a. pulse amplification
    b. time-gain compensation (TGC)
    c. compression
    d. registration
    e. pulse repetition frequency (PRF)

14. Which of the following best characterizes M-mode scanning?
    a. moving interfaces presented along one line
    b. moving interfaces presented within an x-y grid
    c. moving interfaces presented one to a line
    d. moving interfaces presented as a gray scale
    e. moving interfaces presented as 3D images

15. The gray scale of a digital image is determined by which computer feature?
    a. bit depth
    b. clock speed
    c. matrix size
    d. RAM capacity
    e. ROM capacity

16. Smoothing, when applied to postprocessing an image, results in
    a. improved spatial resolution.
    b. improved contrast resolution.
    c. improved signal-to-noise ratio.
    d. fewer artifacts.
    e. edge enhancement.

17. The intensity of the transmitted pulse is adjusted by which control?
    a. depth of focus
    b. amplifier power
    c. receiver gain
    d. time-gain compensation (TGC)
    e. duty factor (DF)

18. The piezoelectric effect converts a pressure pulse to what kind of energy?
    a. light
    b. heat
    c. electrical
    d. mechanical
    e. electromagnetic

19. Which of the following are naturally occurring piezoelectric crystals?

    1. quartz
    2. Rochelle salt
    3. tourmaline
    4. lead zirconate titanate

    a. Only 1, 2, and 3 are correct.
    b. Only 1 and 3 are correct.
    c. Only 2 and 4 are correct.
    d. Only 4 is correct.
    e. All are correct.

20. Which part of the transducer controls ringdown?

    a. radio frequency insulation
    b. matching layer
    c. connectors
    d. backing material
    e. piezoelectric crystal

21. Which of the following improves when the number of realtime scan lines is increased?

    a. energy resolution
    b. axial resolution
    c. lateral resolution
    d. temporal resolution
    e. contrast resolution

22. The center frequency divided by the bandwidth is

    a. duty factor (DF).
    b. Q value.
    c. impedance.
    d. intensity.
    e. power.

23. What is the process of varying the excitation of transducer crystals to form a realtime pulse?

    a. amplification
    b. apodization
    c. registration
    d. misregistration
    e. modulation

24. The width of a realtime ultrasound beam perpendicular to the in-plane axis, commonly called slice thickness, is determined by

    1. acoustic intensity.
    2. acoustic lens.
    3. matrix size.
    4. beam width.

    a. Only 1, 2, and 3 are correct.
    b. Only 1 and 3 are correct.
    c. Only 2 and 4 are correct.
    d. Only 4 is correct.
    e. All are correct.

25. **How does the ultrasonographer control realtime frame rate (FR)?**
    a. pulse amplification
    b. time-gain compensation (TGC)
    c. compression
    d. scan depth
    e. pulse repetition range

26. **When each realtime frame has 180 lines at a rate of 30 frames per second, what is the maximum depth of the image?**
    a. 8 cm
    b. 16 cm
    c. 20 cm
    d. 28 cm
    e. 32 cm

27. **What is the frame rate (FR) for commercial television?**
    a. 16 frames per second
    b. 30 frames per second
    c. 60 frames per second
    d. 90 frames per second
    e. 120 frames per second

28. **What is the number of lines in a commercial television image?**
    a. 256
    b. 512
    c. 525
    d. 825
    e. 1000

29. **Realtime scanning excels as compared with compound B-mode imaging in its**
    a. axial resolution.
    b. lateral resolution.
    c. contrast resolution.
    d. temporal resolution.
    e. energy resolution.

30. **With an annular array, beam steering is done**
    a. by annular delay.
    b. by phased delay.
    c. by mechanical delay.
    d. with acoustic lenses.
    e. with acoustic mirrors.

31. **With a single-element transducer, the beam is focused by**
    a. electronic delay.
    b. curving the crystal.
    c. changing the pulse repetition frequency (PRF).
    d. changing the spatial pulse length (SPL).
    e. changing the Q value.

32. **When referring to a transducer, to what does the one-quarter wavelength refer?**
    a. damping material
    b. matching layer
    c. piezoelectric crystal diameter
    d. piezoelectric crystal thickness
    e. window

33. When the monitor is continually refreshed by a fixed image, the process is called
    a. average frame.
    b. frame averaging.
    c. frame integration.
    d. frame registration.
    e. freeze frame.

34. Realtime imaging with a linear phased array is accomplished by
    a. electronic delay.
    b. sequential activation.
    c. segmental activation.
    d. mechanical means.
    e. acoustic lenses.

35. The fidelity of realtime imaging is determined principally by the
    a. spatial pulse length (SPL).
    b. pulse duration (PD).
    c. field of view (FOV).
    d. frequency.
    e. frame rate (FR).

36. An M-mode scan provides information about interface
    1. depth.
    2. echo intensity.
    3. velocity.
    4. scattering.

    a. Only 1, 2, and 3 are correct.
    b. Only 1 and 3 are correct.
    c. Only 2 and 4 are correct.
    d. Only 4 is correct.
    e. All are correct.

37. During realtime imaging, if the line density (LD) is halved, what happens to maximum frame rate (FR)?
    a. it is reduced to one-fourth
    b. it is halved
    c. no change
    d. it is doubled
    e. it is increased four times

38. Which operator control varies echo amplitude as a function of depth in the patient?
    a. compression
    b. amplification
    c. enveloping
    d. time-gain compensation (TGC)
    e. range signal gating

39. Realtime imaging with a phased-array transducer produces a sector scan image as large as
    a. 30°.
    b. 60°.
    c. 90°.
    d. 120°.
    e. 150°.

40. When a realtime linear-array transducer is used in the multifocus mode, which of the following is reduced?

    a. spatial pulse length (SPL)
    b. pulse duration (PD)
    c. pulse repetition frequency (PRF)
    d. frequency
    e. frame rate (FR)

41. When deeper tissues must be imaged, what technique changes will work?

    a. reduce frequency
    b. increase frequency
    c. reduce pulse repetition frequency (PRF)
    d. increase pulse repetition frequency (PRF)
    e. increase spatial pulse length (SPL)

42. What is the approximate minimum frame rate (FR) in order for a realtime image to be flicker-free?

    a. 10 frames per second
    b. 20 frames per second
    c. 30 frames per second
    d. 40 frames per second
    e. 50 frames per second

43. The operating frequency of an ultrasound imager depends principally on the

    a. pulse programmer.
    b. pulse shaper.
    c. crystal diameter.
    d. crystal thickness.
    e. matching layer.

44. When echoes are rejected by a receiver because they are not sufficiently intense, it is because the

    a. transmitted pulse was improperly shaped.
    b. transmitted pulse was too weak.
    c. dynamic range was too narrow.
    d. sensitivity level was not reached.
    e. threshold level was not reached.

45. Echo dynamic range reduction in gray-scale imagers is accomplished through

    a. time-gain control.
    b. rejection.
    c. comparison.
    d. compression.
    e. enveloping.

46. The most commonly employed scan converter is based on which technology?

    a. analog
    b. bistable
    c. digital
    d. gray scale
    e. quadratic

47. Which characteristic of an imaging system describes its ability to detect and display very weak echoes?

    a. accuracy
    b. compression
    c. precision
    d. reproducibility
    e. sensitivity

48. Which of the following image shapes is produced by a linear-array realtime imager?

    a.   b.   c.

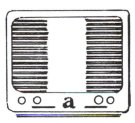 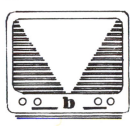 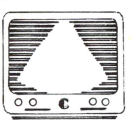

    d.   e.

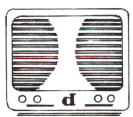 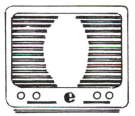

49. What determines the power of an ultrasound beam?

    a. the area of the face of the transducer
    b. the thickness of the piezoelectric crystal
    c. the voltage applied by the pulser
    d. the gain slope of the time-gain compensation (TGC)
    e. the amplification gain of the receiver

50. The difference between the weakest and the strongest echo detected is the

    a. amplification gain.
    b. dynamic range.
    c. gray scale.
    d. rejection scale.
    e. time-gain scale.

51. Which of the following are synthetic piezoelectric crystals?

    1. lead zirconate titanate
    2. barium titanate
    3. lithium sulfate
    4. lead metaniobate

    a. Only 1, 2, and 3 are correct.
    b. Only 1 and 3 are correct.
    c. Only 2 and 4 are correct.
    d. Only 4 is correct.
    e. All are correct.

52. **The piezoelectric effect converts an electric signal to what kind of energy?**
    a. light
    b. heat
    c. electrical
    d. mechanical
    e. electromagnetic

53. **Damping material incorporated into a pulse echo (PE) transducer will**
    1. improve axial resolution.
    2. shorten spatial pulse length (SPL).
    3. reduce pulse duration (PD).
    4. increase Q value.

    a. Only 1, 2, and 3 are correct.
    b. Only 1 and 3 are correct.
    c. Only 2 and 4 are correct.
    d. Only 4 is correct.
    e. All are correct.

54. **Which of the following can be used to couple the transducer to the skin?**
    1. air
    2. aqueous gel
    3. barium sulfate
    4. water

    a. Only 1, 2, and 3 are correct.
    b. Only 1 and 3 are correct.
    c. Only 2 and 4 are correct.
    d. Only 4 is correct.
    e. All are correct.

55. **On an A-mode display, the height of a spike represents**
    a. half the distance to the interface.
    b. the distance to the interface.
    c. twice the distance to the interface.
    d. echo width.
    e. echo intensity.

56. **Which of the following affects the amplification of echoes?**
    1. time-gain compensation (TGC)
    2. balance
    3. compression
    4. output intensity

    a. Only 1, 2, and 3 are correct.
    b. Only 1 and 3 are correct.
    c. Only 2 and 4 are correct.
    d. Only 4 is correct.
    e. All are correct.

57. **Compression adjustment on the receiver affects**
    a. balance.
    b. dynamic range.
    c. intensity.
    d. slope.
    e. time-gain compensation (TGC).

58. In general, which type of resolution is best for complex B-mode imaging?

    a. axial resolution
    b. contrast resolution
    c. energy resolution
    d. lateral resolution
    e. temporal resolution

59. The typical pulse repetition frequency (PRF) for pulse echo (PE) imaging is

    a. 10 Hz.
    b. 100 Hz.
    c. 1 kHz.
    d. 10 kHz.
    e. 100 kHz.

60. The B in B-mode imaging stands for

    a. beam.
    b. binary.
    c. bistable.
    d. bone.
    e. brightness.

61. Which is the most common piezoelectric material?

    a. barium sulfate
    b. barium titanate
    c. quartz
    d. lead metaniobate
    e. lead zirconate titanate

62. Which of the following are sonographer-adjustable?

    1. amplification
    2. compression
    3. rejection
    4. demodulation

    a. Only 1, 2, and 3 are correct.
    b. Only 1 and 3 are correct.
    c. Only 2 and 4 are correct.
    d. Only 4 is correct.
    e. All are correct.

63. What is the gray-scale range of a five-bit digital scan converter?

    a. 16 shades   d. 128 shades
    b. 32 shades   e. 256 shades
    c. 64 shades

64. The receiver does the following.

    a. modulation, sonification, compensation, compression
    b. modulation, demodulation, compression, rejection
    c. sonification, modulation, compensation, compression
    d. amplification, compensation, compression, rejection
    e. amplification, sonification, compression, rejection

65. The ratio of transmitted pulse intensity to echo intensity can be expressed as
   a. enhancement.
   b. compression.
   c. gain.
   d. modulation.
   e. time-gain compensation (TGC).

66. Which of the following is improved when the realtime spatial pulse length (SPL) is reduced?
   a. energy resolution
   b. axial resolution
   c. lateral resolution
   d. temporal resolution
   e. contrast resolution

67. Time-gain compensation (TGC) is necessary to correct for
   a. attenuation.
   b. dynamic range.
   c. Q value.
   d. reflection.
   e. refraction.

68. What is the gray-scale resolution of a realtime imager having a 70-dB dynamic range and a six-bit digital scan converter?
   a. 0.9 dB/gray level
   b. 1.1 dB/gray level
   c. 2.2 dB/gray level
   d. 2.6 dB/gray level
   e. 3.1 dB/gray level

69. The type of transducer that is designed for electronic focusing and mechanical beam steering is the
   a. annular array.
   b. B-mode imager.
   c. color-flow imaging.
   d. linear array.
   e. phased array.

70. Which of the following image shapes is produced by a phased-array realtime imager?

a.

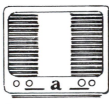

b.

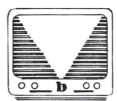

c.

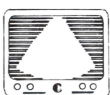

d.

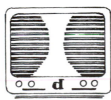

e.

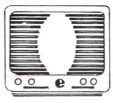

71. In this rendition of a time-gain compensation (TGC) curve, which letter indicates delay?

    a. A   c. C   e. E
    b. B   d. D

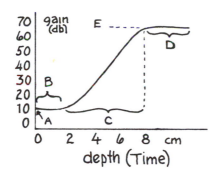

72. What is the approximate frame rate (FR) below which flicker will be apparent?

    a. 8   c. 32   e 128
    b. 16   d. 64

73. Which of the following represents M-mode?

    a.   b.   c.   d.   e.

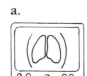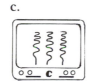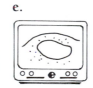

74. An ultrasound imager that can detect weak echoes easily is said to have good

    a. accuracy.   c. precision.   e. sensitivity.
    b. latitude.   d. resolution.

75. A mode stands for

    a. action.   c. amplitude.   e. axial.
    b. alternate.   d. average.

76. In this rendition of a time-gain compensation (TGC) curve, which letter indicates near gain?

    a. A   c. C   e. E
    b. B   d. D

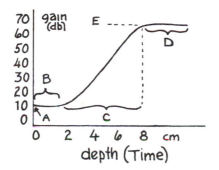

77. Which of the following represents A-mode?

a.
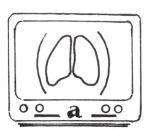

b.
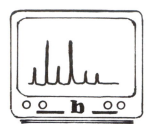

c.
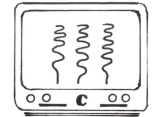

d.
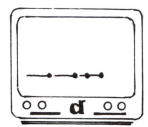

e.
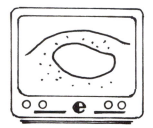

78. Bistable is a term that refers to

    a. electronic drift.
    b. transducer drift.
    c. black and white.
    d. gray scale.
    e. motion.

79. The number of shades of gray between black and white is called

    a. bistable.
    b. bit range.
    c. damping.
    d. dynamic range.
    e. multistable.

80. One method for reducing spatial pulse length (SPL) is

    a. compression.
    b. damping.
    c. enhancement.
    d. shadowing
    e. time-gain compensation (TGC).

81. Intensities employed in ultrasound imaging include

    1. SATA = 100 mW/cm^2 to 1000 mW/cm^2.
    2. SATA = 500 mW/cm^2 to 5000 mW/cm^2.
    3. 10 mW/mW.
    4. SPTA = 2 mW/cm^2 to 500 mW/cm^2.

    a. Only 1, 2, and 3 are correct.
    b. Only 1 and 3 are correct.
    c. Only 2 and 4 are correct.
    d. Only 4 is correct.
    e. All are correct.

82. **Which transducer would be most helpful when imaging tissue within 2 cm of the skin?**

    a. 2 MHz, short focus
    b. 2 MHz, long focus
    c. 2 MHz, variable focus
    d. 5 MHz, short focus
    e. 5 MHz, long focus

83. **The piezoelectric crystal is usually made of**

    a. aluminum (Al).
    b. calcium tungstate (Ca WO4).
    c. lead zirconate titanate (Pb ZT).
    d. lead oxide (Pb O).
    e. lithium fluoride (Li F).

84. **What is the approximate number of gray levels that the eye can distinguish?**

    a. 8   d. 64
    b. 16   e. 128
    c. 32

85. **Which of the following represents B-mode?**

    a.   b.   c.

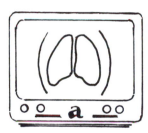 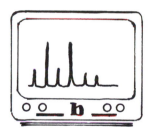 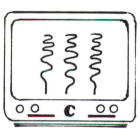

    d.   e.

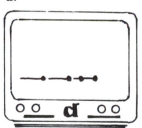 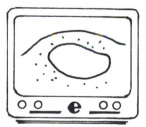

86. **Most current digital ultrasound imagers display what matrix size and dynamic range?**

    a. 128 × 128, four bit
    b. 128 × 128, six bit
    c. 256 × 256, four bit
    d. 256 × 256, six bit
    e. 512 × 512, six bit

87. **Realtime ultrasound has most in common with**

    a. fluoroscopy.   d. SPECT.
    b. MRI.   e. spiral CT.
    c. radiography.

88. Compression occurs in the
    a. amplifier.
    b. pulse programmer.
    c. receiver.
    d. transducer.
    e. transmitter.

89. Rejection occurs in the
    a. amplifier.
    b. pulse programmer.
    c. receiver.
    d. transducer.
    e. transmitter.

90. Lead zirconate titanate is also called
    a. lithionate.   d. quartz.
    b. $PbWO_4$.   e. TLD.
    c. PZT-5.

91. Which of the following have found use in acoustic lenses for beam shaping?
    1. aluminum
    2. lead zirconate titanate
    3. plastic
    4. glass
    a. Only 1, 2, and 3 are correct.
    b. Only 1 and 3 are correct.
    c. Only 2 and 4 are correct.
    d. Only 4 is correct.
    e. All are correct.

92. Which of the following describes regions of the time-gain compensation (TGC) curve?
    1. delay   3. knee
    2. slope   4. far gain
    a. Only 1, 2, and 3 are correct.
    b. Only 1 and 3 are correct.
    c. Only 2 and 4 are correct.
    d. Only 4 is correct.
    e. All are correct.

93. Which of the following is the approximate range of pulse repetition frequency (PRF)?
    a. 1 to 10 Hz
    b. 5 to 50 Hz
    c. 10 to 100 Hz
    d. 500 to 5000 Hz
    e. 100 to 1000 Hz

94. The effects of ultrasound attenuation are corrected by
    a. compression circuit.
    b. demodulator.
    c. frequency analyzer.
    d. time-gain compensation (TGC).
    e. rejection circuit.

95. Operating frequency is determined principally by the
    a. crystal diameter.
    b. crystal thickness.
    c. duty cycle.
    d. pulse programmer.
    e. transducer Q value.

96. Fourier transformation of an echo, signal intensity vs. time, will result in
    a. frequency vs. time.
    b. frequency vs. wavelength.
    c. signal intensity vs. frequency.
    d. signal intensity vs. wavelength.
    e. wavelength vs. time.

97. The digital scan converter is essentially a/an
    a. audio receiver.
    b. cathode ray tube (CRT).
    c. computer.
    d. television.
    e. video receiver.

98. Reducing the angle of a sector scanner will
    a. improve image resolution.
    b. increase frame rate (FR).
    c. increase image time.
    d. reduce line density (LD).
    e. reduce pulse repetition frequency (PRF).

99. Which of the following represents linear scanning?

a.

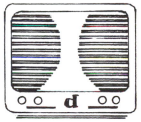

b.

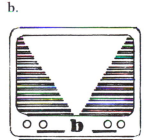

c.

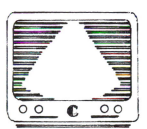

d.

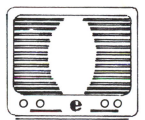

e.

100. Adjusting impedance to affect reduced reflection is the process of
    a. compensating.
    b. compressing.
    c. damping.
    d. demodulating.
    e. matching.

101. What is it called when the piezoelectric crystal continues to vibrate after excitation?

    a. activation
    b. backing
    c. collapsing
    d. damping
    e. ringdown

102. The transducer produces ultrasound using

    a. the photoelectric effect.
    b. liquid crystals.
    c. the piezoelectric effect.
    d. the transducer effect.
    e. Snell's law.

103. Which transducer would be most helpful when imaging tissue beyond 4 cm depth?

    a. 2 MHz, short focus
    b. 2 MHz, long focus
    c. 2 MHz, variable focus
    d. 5 MHz, short focus
    e. 5 MHz, long focus

104. Which of the following is a component of a pulse echo (PE) ultrasound transducer?

    1. antiscatter material
    2. matching layer
    3. gadolinium oxysulfide
    4. backing material

    a. Only 1, 2, and 3 are correct.
    b. Only 1 and 3 are correct.
    c. Only 2 and 4 are correct.
    d. Only 4 is correct.
    e. All are correct.

105. A pulse echo (PE) imager emits a pulse 3 μs long followed by a 497 μs dead time. What is the pulse repetition frequency (PRF)?

    a. 1 kHz
    b. 2 kHz
    c. 3 kHz
    d. 3 μs
    e. 500 μs

106. The thickness of a piezoelectric crystal is closest to

    a. 1 μm.
    b. 10 μm.
    c. 100 μm.
    d. 1000 μm.
    e. 10,000 μm.

107. The active element of an ultrasound transducer converts

    1. wavelength into frequency.
    2. power into intensity.
    3. mechanical energy into sound energy.
    4. electric energy into mechanical energy.

    a. Only 1, 2, and 3 are correct.
    b. Only 1 and 3 are correct.
    c. Only 2 and 4 are correct.
    d. Only 4 is correct.
    e. All are correct.

108. In fabricating a pulse echo (PE) transducer, backing material is used to

    a. attach maximum skin coupling.
    b. attach electrodes.
    c. enhance reverberation.
    d. increase intensity.
    e. improve axial resolution.

109. A necessary condition to produce diagnostic ultrasound echoes is

    a. sound frequency of 1 to 15 mHz.
    b. sound wavelength less than 1 mm.
    c. differences of acoustic impedance.
    d. differences in atomic number.
    e. differences in mass density.

110. When operating in the M mode, M stands, for

    a. magnitude.
    b. major.
    c. maximum.
    d. module.
    e. motion.

111. Of the number techniques for displaying an ultrasound signal,

    a. abdominal imaging is usually done in realtime.
    b. echocardiography usually employs B mode.
    c. A mode is most often used in obstetrics.
    d. Doppler mode produces the best image.
    e. M mode is used when echoes are weak.

112. In pulse echo (PE) A mode, which of the following represents the distance between blips?

    a. velocity $\times$ one-quarter time to interface
    b. velocity $\times$ one-half time to interface
    c. velocity $\times$ time to interface
    d. velocity $\times$ two times to interface
    e. velocity $\times$ four times to interface

113. **Which of the following represents a phased-array sector scan?**

a.

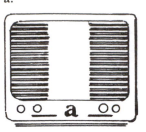

b.

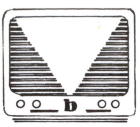

c.

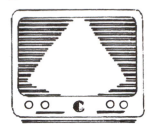

d.

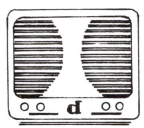

e.

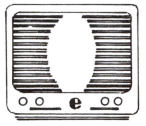

114. **In B-mode imaging, the B stands for**

    a. bistable.
    b. body.
    c. bone.
    d. brightness.
    e. bulk.

115. **Realtime ultrasound imaging**

    a. has better lateral resolution than B mode.
    b. is accomplished with a single crystal.
    c. is accomplished with a linear array of crystals.
    d. requires several transducers if a phased array is used.
    e. must be digital.

116. **In this rendition of a time-gain compensation (TGC) curve, which letter indicates far gain?**

    a. A   **d.** D
    b. B   **e.** E
    c. C

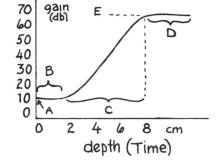

117. **B-mode gray-scale imaging is possible principally because of the**

    a. microprocessor.
    b. A/D converter.
    c. D/A converter.
    d. scan converter.
    e. laser camera.

Doppler Ultrasound

- The Doppler effect was first described by Austrian physicist Christian Doppler in 1848.

- The Doppler effect is the apparent change in frequency in either sound or light due to the motion of either the source or the receiver.

- The change in pitch of the sound of a train's whistle that is heard as it passes is an example of the Doppler effect.

- The fact that there are more red-shift stars than blue-shift stars, a Doppler effect, led to the knowledge that our universe is expanding.

- The application of the Doppler effect in ultrasound is directed principally to naturally moving tissues, such as cardiac membranes and blood.

- There are three types of Doppler instruments: continuous-wave (CW), pulse echo (PE), and color flow.

- Commonly used frequencies are 2 to 10 MHz.

- Commonly used intensities are 0.2 to 2000 mW/cm^2.

- Doppler examination with realtime imaging and continuous-wave and/or pulse echo is available.

THE DOPPLER EQUATION

- The **Doppler shift frequency** (F_D) is the difference between the transmitted frequency (F_T) and that reflected from a moving interface (F_R).

- If the tissue is moving toward the transducer, F_R will be higher than F_T, resulting in a positive F_D. In color-flow Doppler, this would usually be rendered as blue.

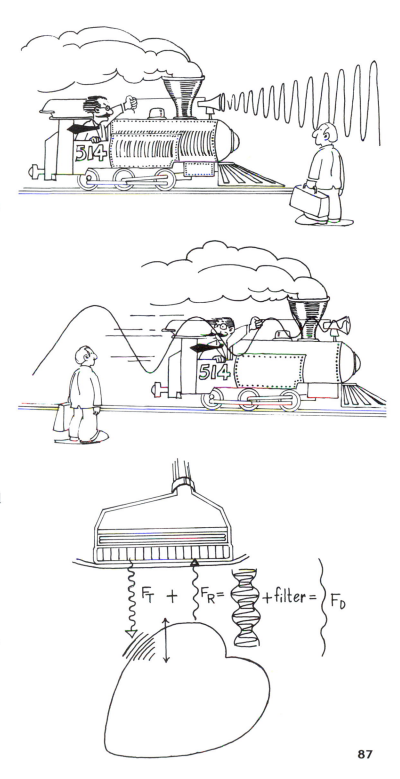

$$F_T + F_R = \text{filter} = F_D$$

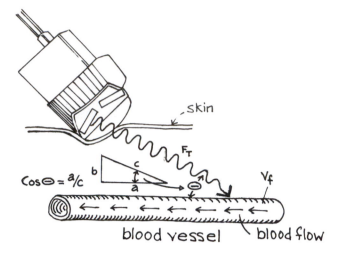

$$\text{Cos}\,\ominus = a/c$$

skin

blood vessel   blood flow

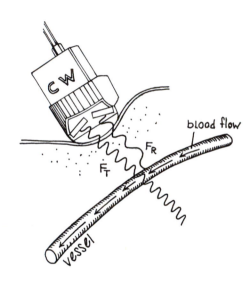

blood flow

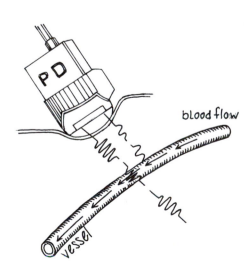

blood flow

- If the interface is moving away from the transducer, F_R will be less than F_T resulting in a negative F_D. In color flow Doppler, this is usually rendered as red.

- The Doppler shift frequency is also the product of twice the transmitted frequency times the velocity of the interface divided by the velocity of ultrasound in tissue.

- In medical imaging, interface velocity is usually such that F_D is in the audible range, so that one can listen to sound characteristics of the interface velocity.

THE DOPPLER ANGLE

- The value of the reflected frequency changes as a function of the **Doppler angle**.

- The Doppler angle is that between the central axis of the ultrasound beam and the direction of movement of tissue, usually flowing blood.

- The Doppler shift frequency is reduced by the cosine of the Doppler angle.

- The optimum Doppler angle is 30° to 60°.

- Doppler angles less than 30° result in loss of signal due to refraction.

- Doppler angles greater than 60° result in loss of signal because the Doppler shift frequency is too small.

- At a Doppler angle of 90°, the Doppler shift frequency is zero.

- An error in Doppler angle estimation can result in a very large error in velocity estimation.

- Doppler shift frequencies usually range from approximately 200 Hz to 15 kHz and thus are in the audible range.

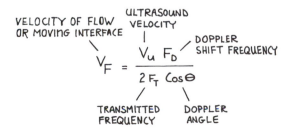

$$V_F = \frac{V_u \; F_D}{2\, F_T \; \text{Cos}\,\ominus}$$

VELOCITY OF FLOW OR MOVING INTERFACE — ULTRASOUND VELOCITY — DOPPLER SHIFT FREQUENCY — TRANSMITTED FREQUENCY — DOPPLER ANGLE

- Continuous-wave (CW) Doppler instruments contain two transducers—one for transmission and the other for echo reception.

- CW Doppler has a duty factor of 1.

- Pulse echo Doppler has a single transducer element.

- Doppler combined with realtime imaging requires two transducers and is called **duplex imaging**.

- The principal disadvantage to CW Doppler is that all moving tissues within the sensitive depth of the transducer will be detected. This superposition of signals makes analysis more difficult.

- Pulse echo Doppler allows analysis of multiple vessels.

- Pulse echo Doppler allows analysis of vessels at different depths.

- Color-flow imaging combines B-mode imaging and CW Doppler signal processing.

- Color-flow imaging usually codes flow away from the transducer red and that toward the transducer blue; however, the opposite is employed by some vendors.

- Color intensity in color-flow imaging increases with increasing flow.

- Color-flow imagers measure frequency and calculate velocity from the Doppler equation.

- Pulse echo Doppler imagers allow both imaging and flow analysis.

- **Range gating** is the electronic window of pulse Doppler systems that allow signal analysis from a section of tissue at a given depth.

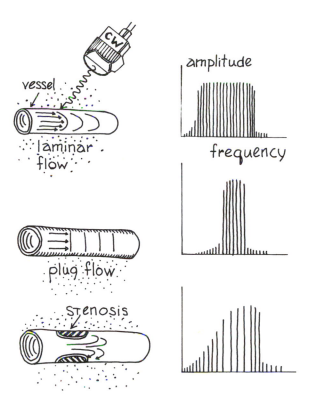

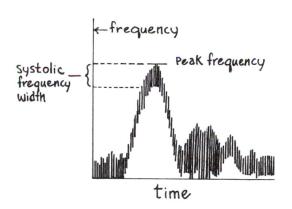

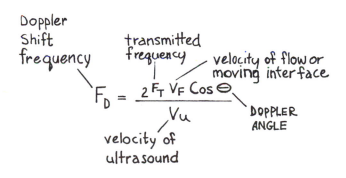

$$F_D = \frac{2 F_T V_F \cos \Theta}{V_u}$$

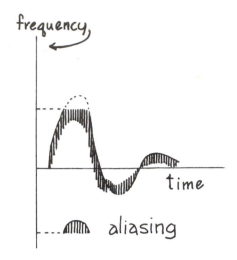

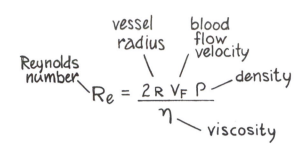

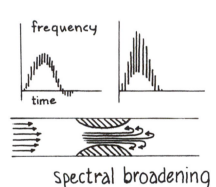

spectral broadening

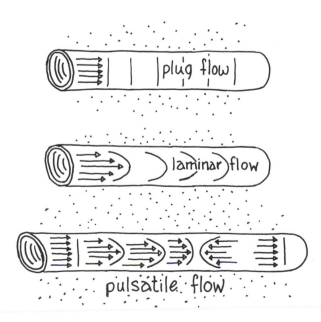

- The velocity of ultrasound in blood is 1580 m/s.

- Blood has low ultrasound attenuation (approximately 0.2 dB/cm/MHz); therefore cardiac imaging requires less intensity.

- Red blood cells are small, approximately 8 μm in diameter, and are therefore diffuse reflectors.

- There is never a single Doppler shift frequency; rather, the variation in blood velocity results in a spectrum of frequencies.

- The Doppler frequency spectrum is a plot of the amplitude of the various frequencies in the Doppler echo vs. frequency.

- The realtime Doppler spectrum is a plot of frequency vs. time.

- It is the realtime Doppler spectrum that can exhibit the aliasing artifact.

- Spectral analysis of Doppler signals from flowing blood allows the diagnosis of thrombosis, stenosis, and other vascular disorders.

- **Spectral broadening** occurs because of disorganized flow.

- Fast Fourier transformation of Doppler shift frequencies—blood cell velocities—can be displayed as function of time, the realtime Doppler spectrum.

- The Reynolds number (Re) predicts turbulent flow.

- The display of the spectrum of blood velocity allows analysis of the type of blood flow.

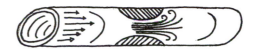

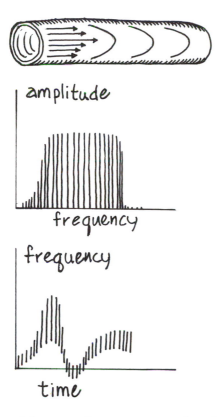

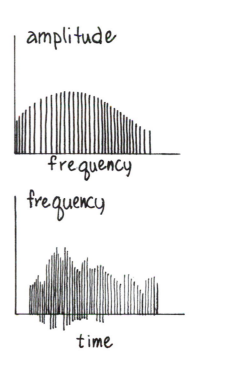

- Normal **laminar flow** is associated with venous circulation in healthy straight vessels.

- Laminar flow produces a narrow range of velocities and therefore a narrow bandwidth in the Doppler shift spectrum.

- The laminar flow pattern is called **parabolic** because the blood flows in concentric layers, moving parallel with the vessel wall.

- Arterial blood flow during systole is **plug flow**; that is, all with the same velocity.

- Increased flow rates at a stenosis site produce a wider range of velocities and therefore spectral broadening.

- **Spectral broadening** indicates peripheral vascular disease.

- Negative frequency values in spectrum analysis indicate turbulence and eddy currents downstream from a stenosis.

- Of the many numerical indices obtained from the spectrum waveform, two are particularly helpful—the pulsatility index and the resistance index.

- High values of either of these indices indicate vascular disease.

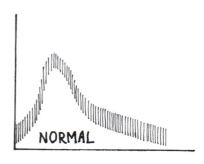

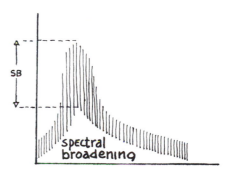

- The **pulsatility index** is the peak-to-peak waveform value divided by the mean.

- The **resistance index** is the peak systole value minus the end diastole value divided by the peak systole value.

- The resistance index is also known as **Pourcelot's index.**

- Blood flow velocity can be estimated using the Doppler equation.

- Blood volume flow can be estimated using the Doppler equation and the cross section of the vessel.

Chapter 6 Review Questions

1. The operating frequency is 2.25 MHz. What is the approximate Doppler shift frequency at a 0° angle with blood having velocity of 30 cm/s?

   a. 360 Hz   d. 720 Hz
   b. 430 Hz   e. 860 Hz
   c. 550 Hz

2. In a pulsed-wave Doppler spectrum, what does the horizontal axis measure?

   a. frequency
   b. time
   c. velocity
   d. depth
   e. intensity

3. Which of the following can be determined with Doppler imaging regarding a moving interface?

   1. depth   3. velocity
   2. direction   4. power

   a. Only 1, 2, and 3 are correct.
   b. Only 1 and 3 are correct.
   c. Only 2 and 4 are correct.
   d. Only 4 is correct.
   e. All are correct.

4. What is the Doppler shift frequency in soft tissue if a 2.25 MHz transducer is directed at 30° to 15 cm/s interface?

   a. 378 Hz   d. 3462 Hz
   b. 517 Hz   e. 9077 Hz
   c. 1115 Hz

5. What is the velocity of a moving soft tissue interface if a Doppler shift frequency of 2000 Hz is detected with a 2.25 MHz transducer at a 20° angle to the interface?

   a. 13 m/s
   b. 27 m/s
   c. 67 m/s
   d. 73 m/s
   e. 91 m/s

6. What term is applied to color-flow image detection?

   a. registration
   b. misregistration
   c. fast Fourier transformation
   d. autocorrelation
   e. enveloping

7. When transducer frequency is reduced, what happens to the Doppler shift frequency of a moving tissue?

   a. it decreases
   b. it remains the same
   c. it increases
   d. it increases or decreases, depending on the direction of motion
   e. it increases or decreases, depending on tissue type

8. What type of ultrasound imager has both realtime and Doppler capacity?

   a. A mode
   b. B mode
   c. C mode
   d. M mode
   e. color-flow imaging

9. Blood flow is inversely proportional to

   a. mass density.
   b. viscosity.
   c. vessel radius.
   d. blood pressure.
   e. vessel length.

10. In what range will the Doppler shift frequency of blood normally be found?

    a. subsonic
    b. audible
    c. ultrasonic
    d. hypersonic
    e. hyposonic

11. What is the velocity of blood if the Doppler shift frequency is 2 KHz measured at a 45° angle with a 2.25 MHz transducer?

    a. 4.2 cm/s
    b. 9.9 cm/s
    c. 12 cm/s
    d. 21 cm/s
    e. 33 cm/s

12. If peak flow through the aortic valve is 4 m/s, what is the pressure gradient?
    a. 4 mmHg
    b. 8 mmHg
    c. 16 mmHg
    d. 32 mmHg
    e. 64 mmHg

13. The temporal resolution of color-flow imaging can be improved with a/an
    a. duplex scanner.
    b. synchronous scanner.
    c. iteration function.
    d. autocorrelation function.
    e. fast Fourier transform.

14. As the ultrasonographer positions a transesophageal probe closer to the heart, which of the following can be increased?
    1. frame rate (FR)
    2. output intensity
    3. image lines
    4. output power

    a. Only 1, 2, and 3 are correct.
    b. Only 1 and 3 are correct.
    c. Only 2 and 4 are correct.
    d. Only 4 is correct.
    e. All are correct.

15. Cardiac ejection fraction is defined as the fractional change in left ventricular volume
    a. during diastole.
    b. during systole.
    c. between diastole and systole.
    d. between stress and rest.
    e. at maximum heart rate.

16. In color-flow imaging, turbulent flow appears
    a. as a sharp boundary.
    b. as a smooth boundary.
    c. as a mosaic.
    d. uniform.
    e. striated.

17. In cardiac imaging, axial resolution can be improved by
    a. increasing pulse duration (PD).
    b. increasing frequency.
    c. reducing line density (LD).
    d. reducing pulse repetition rate (PRR).
    e. using a smaller transducer.

18. Blood flow is proportional to the fourth power of
    a. optical density.
    b. mass density.
    c. vessel radius.
    d. pressure gradient.
    e. viscosity.

19. Laminar flow is best described by
    a. layered flow.
    b. uniform flow.
    c. no flow.
    d. high velocity.
    e. low velocity.

20. In color-flow Doppler imaging, increasing packet size provides a better estimate of
    a. lateral resolution.
    b. axial resolution.
    c. temporal resolution.
    d. velocity.
    e. intensity.

21. In a pulsed-wave Doppler spectrum, what does the vertical axis measure?
    a. frequency
    b. time
    c. velocity
    d. depth
    e. intensity

22. The operating frequency is 2.25 MHz. What is the Doppler shift frequency if the angle with 30 cm/s flowing blood is 30°?
    a. 370 Hz   d. 980 Hz
    b. 740 Hz   e. 1720 Hz
    c. 860 Hz

23. Relative to soft tissue, the velocity of sound in blood is approximately
    a. half as slow.
    b. slightly slower.
    c. the same.
    d. slightly faster.
    e. twice as fast.

24. How does the intensity of echoes from red blood cells compare with that from a soft tissue interface?
    a. much weaker
    b. slightly weaker
    c. about the same
    d. slightly stronger
    e. much stronger

25. The velocity of blood flow is directly proportional to
    a. blood viscosity.
    b. vessel diameter.
    c. vessel wall rigidity.
    d. mass density.
    e. differential pressure.

26. **Blood pressure is measured in**

    a. pascals.
    b. atmospheres.
    c. millimeters of mercury.
    d. inches of water.
    e. newtons.

27. **The principle of energy conservation through the entire circulatory system is that of**

    a. Bernoulli.
    b. Boyle.
    c. Charles.
    d. Huygens.
    e. Poisson.

28. **If the hematocrit increases from 42% to 47%, what happens to blood viscosity?**

    a. large decrease
    b. slight decrease
    c. remains the same
    d. slight increase
    e. large increase

29. **Which of the following represents eddy currents?**

    a. A
    b. B
    c. C
    d. D
    e. E

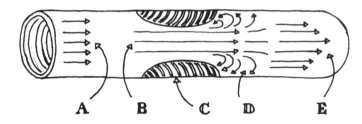

30. **When arteries expand in order to increase blood volume, the process is called**

    a. absorption.
    b. attenuation.
    c. compliance.
    d. impedance.
    e. resistance.

31. **Arterial pulsatile flow is due to**

    a. attenuation.
    b. cardiac contraction.
    c. compliance.
    d. resistance.
    e. pressure differential.

32. **What ultimately restricts blood flow rate?**

    a. aortic valve size
    b. lumen size
    c. mass density
    d. peripheral resistance
    e. viscosity of blood

33. Above what value Reynolds number is turbulent flow indicated?

    a. 0.2
    b. 2
    c. 20
    d. 200
    e. 2000

34. Which of the following measurements of pressure is affected by whether the patient stands or lies down?

    a. differential
    b. Doppler
    c. dynamic
    d. hydrostatic
    e. transient

35. Which of the following represents plug flow?

    a. A
    b. B
    c. C
    d. D
    e. E

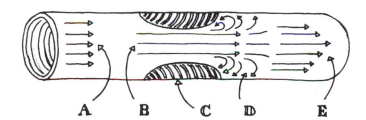

36. Which of the following can occur with pulse Doppler but not normally with continuous-wave (CW) Doppler?

    1. frequency shift
    2. better axial resolution
    3. range data
    4. aliasing

    a. Only 1, 2, and 3 are correct.
    b. Only 1 and 3 are correct.
    c. Only 2 and 4 are correct.
    d. Only 4 is correct.
    e. All are correct.

37. A duplex scanner is one that incorporates

    a. realtime and dead time.
    b. realtime and Doppler.
    c. Doppler and segmental arrays.
    d. segmental and sequential arrays.
    e. Doppler and M-mode.

38. What is the approximate normal peak systolic pressure?

    a. 60 mmHg
    b. 90 mmHg
    c. 120 mmHg
    d. 150 mmHg
    e. 180 mmHg

39. A 2.25 MHz continuous-wave (CW) transducer detects reflected ultrasound at 2.2 MHz. The interface is
    a. moving toward the transducer.
    b. moving away from the transducer.
    c. oscillating.
    d. angulated.
    e. stationary.

40. The weighted sum of frequencies in the power spectrum is the
    a. minimum.
    b. mean.
    c. mode.
    d. median.
    e. maximum.

41. What percent of luminal restriction is required to reduce blood flow significantly?
    a. 10
    b. 40
    c. 70
    d. 90
    e. 99

42. What is the blood velocity profile in the aorta during systole?
    a. laminar
    b. plug
    c. retrograde
    d. smooth
    e. turbulent

43. What is normal cardiac output at rest?
    a. 0.5 L/min
    b. 1.0 L/min
    c. 5 L/min
    d. 10 L/min
    e. 50 L/min

44. Vigorous exercise affects the arteries of the leg by producing
    1. high pulsatile flow.
    2. high laminar flow.
    3. vasoconstriction.
    4. vasodilatation.

    a. Only 1, 2, and 3 are correct.
    b. Only 1 and 3 are correct.
    c. Only 2 and 4 are correct.
    d. Only 4 is correct.
    e. All are correct.

45. The velocity profile of blood changes most markedly
    a. in the capillaries.
    b. from cycle to cycle.
    c. at a bifurcation.
    d. during systole.
    e. during diastole.

46. Continuous-wave (CW) Doppler usually employs a duty cycle of what percent?

a. <1
b. 1 to 5
c. 5 to 10
d. 10 to 25
e. 100

47. Which of the following is most often used for damping material in a continuous-wave (CW) Doppler transducer?

a. air
b. cork
c. epoxy resin
d. rubber
e. tungsten

48. The range of frequencies contained in an echo are measured by

a. the American Institute of Ultrasound in Medicine (AIUM) phantom.
b. energy discrimination.
c. resolution assay.
d. spectrum analysis.
e. temporal analysis.

49. Which of the following represents laminar flow?

a. A
b. B
c. C
d. D
e. E

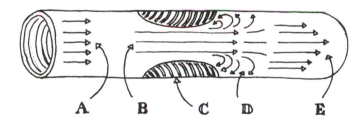

50. Which of the following intensity ranges are used in color-flow imaging?

a. 0.1 to 100 mW/cm^2
b. 0.1 to 500 mW/cm^2
c. 1 to 1000 mW/cm^2
d. 100 to 5000 mW/cm^2
e. 500 to 10,000 mW/cm^2

51. Color-flow imaging can distinguish between positive and negative Doppler frequency shifts. That property is called

a. bidirectional.
b. bistable.
c. demodulated.
d. modulated.
e. polarized.

52. Which of the following angles ($\propto$) between the transducer and blood flow direction will produce the smallest Doppler shift frequency?

a. 5°
b. 30°
c. 45°
d. 60°
e. 85°

53. **When operating in the continuous-wave (CW) Doppler mode,**
    a. one is employing the pulse echo technique.
    b. meaningful information can be obtained only from moving interfaces.
    c. the principal application is the measurement of midline shifts of the brain.
    d. the equipment is more expensive than B-mode imaging.
    e. the Doppler shift frequency (D_F) is usually above 20 kHz.

54. **What is the approximate Doppler shift frequency (D_F) in soft tissue when the transmitted frequency is 3 MHz and the velocity of a perpendicular interface is 10 cm/s?**
    a. 20 Hz
    b. 150 Hz
    c. 390 Hz
    d. 1 MHz
    e. 3 MHz

55. **Which of the following imagers require pulse echo (PE) ultrasound?**
    1. A-mode
    2. B-mode
    3. realtime
    4. Doppler mode

    a. Only 1, 2, and 3 are correct.
    b. Only 1 and 3 are correct.
    c. Only 2 and 4 are correct.
    d. Only 4 is correct.
    e. All are correct.

56. **Which scan image is a sector type?**
    a. linear
    b. phased array
    c. compound B
    d. Doppler
    e. M mode

57. **What is the approximate normal peak diastolic pressure?**
    a. 60 mmHg
    b. 90 mmHg
    c. 120 mmHg
    d. 150 mmHg
    e. 180 mmHg

58. **Which of the following represents turbulent flow?**
    a. A
    b. B
    c. C
    d. D
    e. E

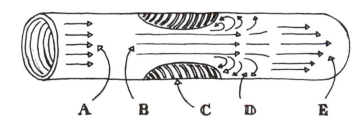

Ultrasound Image Artifacts

- An **artifact** is any unintended signal or information that does not represent the object.

- An **image artifact** is a false feature of an image caused by equipment deficiency, peculiar patient features, patient instability, or image processing defects.

- Ultrasound image artifacts are usually classified according to **reverberation**, **shadowing**, **enhancement**, **displacement**, **distortion**, and **aliasing**.

REVERBERATION

- The reverberation artifact appears as closely spaced interfaces that do not represent actual interfaces.

- The reverberation artifact occurs only when the ultrasound beam is perpendicular to the involved interfaces.

- Occasionally the reverberation artifact will occur inside a mass that appears either cystic or solid.

- A characteristic reverberation artifact is called the **comet tail**.

- Another characteristic artifact is called a **ring-down** artifact.

- Reverberation artifact occurs when an ultrasound beam encounters two highly reflective interfaces that are close to one another.

- Multiple repeating reflections at the interfaces result in false interfaces appearing distal to the true interface.

- Typically, reverberation artifacts occur between transducer and bowel gas, transducer and anterior bladder wall, and the fat layer between skin and muscle.

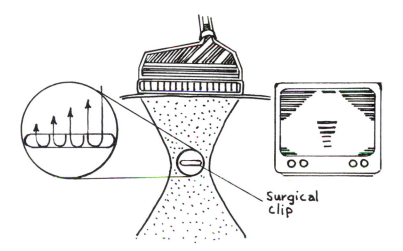

Surgical clip

- Reverberation artifacts can usually be distinguished through anatomy by simply repositioning the transducer so that the beam is not perpendicular to the involved interfaces.

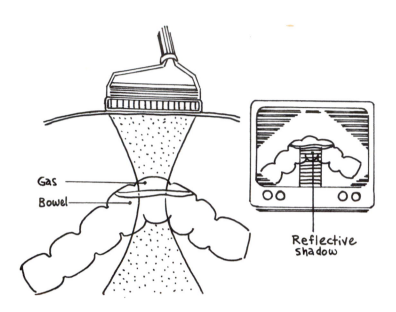

Gas
Bowel
Reflective shadow

SHADOWING

- There are two general types of tissue interfaces—**diffuse reflectors** and **specular reflectors**.

- Diffuse reflectors are rough, irregular tissue interfaces and result in a less intense echo.

- Specular reflectors are smooth tissue interfaces and return strong echoes.

- Specular reflecting interfaces are responsible for the shadowing artifact.

- A specular reflector reflects most of the ultrasound beam, leaving little to interact with deeper tissues.

- The result is no signal and a shadow.

- When the shadowing artifact occurs, deeper tissues important to diagnosis may be absent in the image.

- Shadowing can also result from highly attenuating tissue, such as bowel gas, renal calculi, gallstones, kidney stones, and compact bone.

- Edge shadows can occur at a curved interface, resulting from refraction rather than reflection.

- Edge shadows are a consequence of traversing a curved interface separating tissues that have different ultrasound velocities.

- Sometimes the shadowing artifact can be removed by repositioning the transducer or increasing the far-field time-gain compensation (TGC).

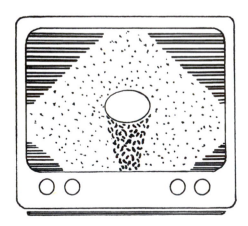

ENHANCEMENT/DISPLACEMENT/ DISTORTION

- **Enhancement** occurs when the TGC is set for soft tissue but another tissue of lower attenuation is in the beam.

- When diagnostic ultrasound passes through less attenuating fluid-filled structures, such as the bladder or a cyst, false amplification produces enhancement of distal tissue because there is increased attenuation in surrounding soft tissue.

- The enhancement artifact is helpful in distinguishing between a solid and a cystic mass.

- **Displacement** occurs when structures in the ultrasound beam are not seen in their true position in the image.

- Side lobes and grating lobes can result in spurious images in the ultrasound image.

- Displacement also occurs when structures outside of the ultrasound beam appear in the image.

- Displacement can be caused by misregistration, a fault of the time/space calipers for an articulated transducer.

- The mirror image sometimes seen on either side of the diaphragm—a strong reflector—is a displacement artifact.

- Misregistration cannot occur in real-time imaging.

- The multipath artifact can appear when a concave specular reflector or multiple oblique interfaces are in the beam.

- Multipath structures appearing in the image are displacement artifacts.

- Refraction can also cause displacement artifacts.

- When the ultrasound beam width varies significantly with depth—e.g., side lobes—object displacement can occur.

- The **distortion** artifact can appear as either geometric distortion or signal intensity distortion.

- Geometric distortion can occur because of changing beam size with depth into the patient.

- Signal intensity distortion occurs when the digital scan converter has too narrow a dynamic range—too few gray levels.

ALIASING

- **Aliasing** is an artifact associated only with Doppler ultrasound.

- When the Doppler shift frequency is not sampled fast enough in a pulsed system, aliasing can occur.

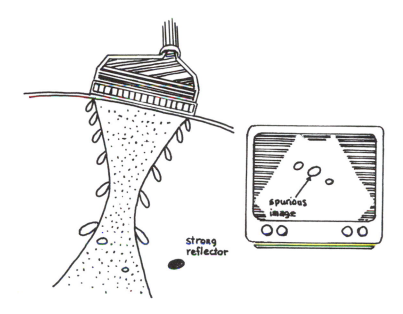

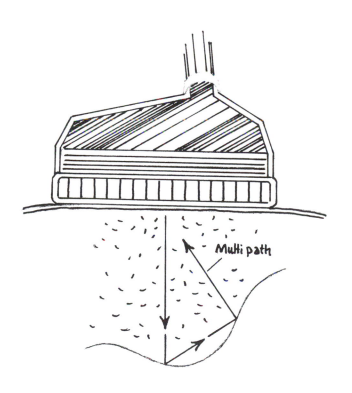

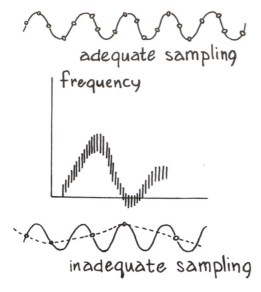

adequate sampling

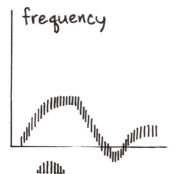

inadequate sampling

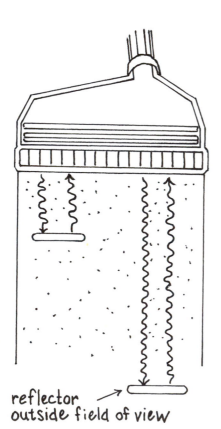

reflector →
outside field of view

- In order to avoid aliasing, one must sample above the Nyquist limit.

- The Nyquist limit requires sampling at least twice in each cycle.

- When the Doppler shift frequency exceeds half the pulse repetition frequency (PRF), aliasing will occur.

- Aliasing can be corrected by increasing the PRF (shorter depth of field) or decreasing the Doppler shift frequency.

- The Doppler shift frequency is reduced by reducing the transmit frequency, bringing the Doppler angle closer to 90°, or providing a reference signal frequency offset.

COLOR-FLOW IMAGING

- Since color-flow imaging combines B mode and Doppler, artifacts associated with both are possible, but three stand out—range ambiguity, aliasing, and soft tissue vibrations.

- **Range ambiguity** occurs principally because of the high frame rates employed and appears as diffuse nonpusatile colors.

- Range ambiguity is an artifact because it indicates flow when none exists.

- Aliasing in color-flow imaging results in the wrapping not only of the frequency spectrum but also of the colors.

- **Vibration** of soft tissues because of patient motion, talking, or turbulent flow can fill a carotid artery with diffuse colors instead of intense flow color.

Chapter 7 Review Questions

1. The aliasing artifact appears
   a. in realtime images.
   b. when using compound B-mode.
   c. with continuous-wave (CW) Doppler.
   d. with pulsed Doppler.
   e. during M-mode examination.

2. A structure that has no echoes and transmits ultrasound with little attenuation is called
   a. anechoic.
   b. echogenic.
   c. hyperechoic.
   d. hypoechoic.
   e. sonolucent.

3. The shadowing artifact
   a. is often observed beyond cystic structures.
   b. occurs most often at high frequency.
   c. is caused by different attenuation of tissues.
   d. results from velocity differences.
   e. results from refraction.

4. During realtime imaging, the ringdown artifact is a result of
   a. resonance in air-filled cavities.
   b. refraction at a tissue interface.
   c. velocity differences.
   d. nonspecular reflection.
   e. refraction.

5. A highly reflective yet small interface can cause what kind of artifact?
   a. ringdown   d. ghost
   b. comet tail   e. aliasing
   c. reverberation

6. When two specular reflectors are close, what is the most likely artifact?
   a. comet tail   d. speckle
   b. ghost   e. aliasing
   c. reverberation

7. Which of the following is most likely to produce a reverberation artifact?
   a. parallel interfaces
   b. long spatial pulse length (SPL)
   c. small angle of incidence
   d. high frequency
   e. smaller transducer size

8. Enhancement occurs because of
   a. weakly attenuating tissue.
   b. strongly attenuating tissue.
   c. Doppler shift.
   d. Huygens' principle.
   e. parallel interfaces.

9. When ultrasound is incident on a curved interface such as fetal skull, an acoustic shadow can result in

   a. comet tail.
   b. edge artifact.
   c. enhancement.
   d. ghost.
   e. scattering.

10. If an image artifact appears as parallel equally spaced lines, the cause is probably

   a. acoustic enhancement.
   b. acoustic shadowing.
   c. multiangle.
   d. refraction.
   e. reverberation.

11. Acoustic enhancement is most likely to occur posterior to a

   a. fetal skull.
   b. calcified mass.
   c. filled urinary bladder.
   d. gallstone.
   e. kidney stone.

12. What can cause false echoes?

   a. absorption
   b. diffraction
   c. rarefaction
   d. reflection
   e. reverberation

13. The mirror-image artifact would most likely be observed near the

   a. diaphragm.
   b. kidney.
   c. lung.
   d. pancreas.
   e. vessel.

14. The comet tail artifact will most likely be observed following an object/tissue interface

   a. of nearly equal acoustic impedance.
   b. of large acoustic impedance mismatch.
   c. that is specular in nature.
   d. that is diffuse in nature.
   e. and very high intensity ultrasound.

15. Echoes that have lower intensity from normal adjacent tissue are called

   a. anechoic.
   b. echogenic.
   c. hyperechoic.
   d. hypoechoic.
   e. sonolucent.

16. Which type of artifact could result from surgical clips, shotgun pellets, or other small metallic bodies?
    a. comet tail
    b. mirror image
    c. multipath
    d. reverberation
    e. ringdown

17. A structure that produces many echoes is called
    a. anechoic.
    b. echogenic.
    c. hyperechoic.
    d. hypoechoic.
    e. sonolucent.

18. Acoustic enhancement occurs when one images a
    a. specular interface.
    b. highly reflective interface.
    c. refractive object.
    d. diffractive object.
    e. weakly attenuating object.

19. The aliasing artifact is due to
    a. undersampling.
    b. intermittent sampling.
    c. inadequate range focusing.
    d. inadequate lateral focusing.
    e. frequency being too low.

20. When a pulse travels multiple times between the transducer and interface, the result may be
    a. aliasing.
    b. enhancement.
    c. multipath artifact.
    d. reverberation.
    e. shadowing.

21. Shadowing occurs because of
    a. weakly attenuating tissue.
    b. strongly attenuation tissue.
    c. Doppler shift.
    d. Huygens' principle.
    e. parallel interfaces.

22. Which of the following could produce a pseudo mass in the image?
    1. mirror image
    2. multipath
    3. side lobe
    4. comet tail

    a. Only 1, 2, and 3 are correct.
    b. Only 1 and 3 are correct.
    c. Only 2 and 4 are correct.
    d. Only 4 is correct.
    e. All are correct.

23. Which of the following may be the cause of acoustic shadowing?
    1. bone/soft tissue interface
    2. gallstones
    3. gas/soft tissue interface
    4. surgical clips

    a. Only 1, 2, and 3 are correct.
    b. Only 1 and 3 are correct.
    c. Only 2 and 4 are correct.
    d. Only 4 is correct.
    e. All are correct.

24. A structure that produces no echoes is called

    a. anechoic.
    b. echogenic.
    c. hyperechoic.
    d. hypoechoic.
    e. sonolucent.

25. Ultrasound images should be presented
    1. from the patient's feet, if transverse.
    2. supine, if transverse.
    3. with the patient's head to the left, if sagittal.
    4. supine, if sagittal.

    a. Only 1, 2, and 3 are correct.
    b. Only 1 and 3 are correct.
    c. Only 2 and 4 are correct.
    d. Only 4 is correct.
    e. All are correct.

26. Which of the following x ray contrast agents will reflect an unacceptable amount of ultrasound?
    1. air (colon)
    2. Hypaque (in intravenous pyelography)
    3. barium sulfate (upper GI)
    4. Telepaque (gallbladder)

    a. Only 1, 2, and 3 are correct.
    b. Only 1 and 3 are correct.
    c. Only 2 and 4 are correct.
    d. Only 4 is correct.
    e. All are correct.

27. When an image artifact appears as an echo increase because of low attenuating overlying tissue, the cause is probably

    a. acoustic enhancement.
    b. acoustic shadowing.
    c. multiangle.
    d. refraction.
    e. reverberation.

28. **Acoustic shadowing is most likely to occur posterior to a**

    a. calcified mass.
    b. fluid-filled object.
    c. gallbladder
    d. prostate gland.
    e. urinary bladder.

29. **Echoes that have higher intensity from normal adjacent tissue are called**

    a. anechoic.
    b. echogenic.
    c. hyperechoic.
    d. hypoechoic.
    e. sonolucent.

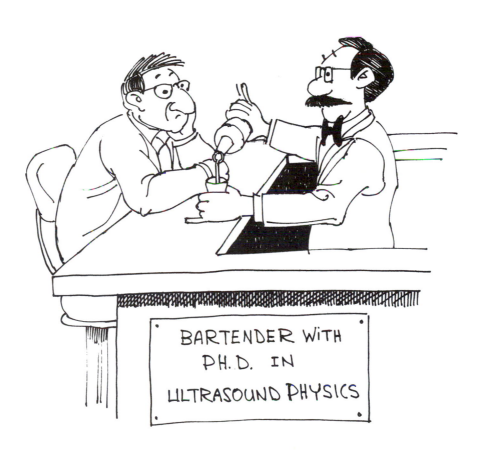

BARTENDER WITH PH.D. IN ULTRASOUND PHYSICS

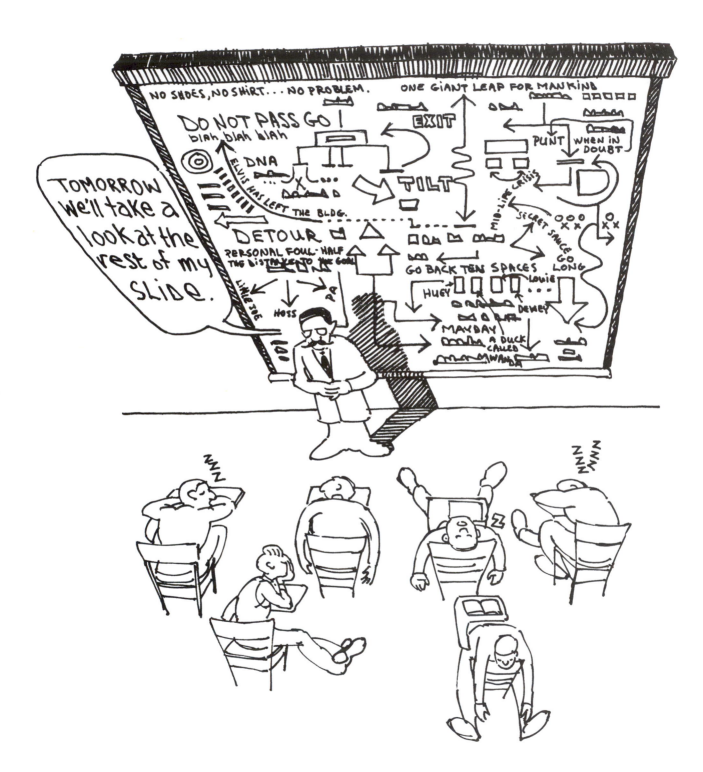

Ultrasound Quality Control

- **Quality assurance** consists of all programs designed to render a diagnostic or therapeutic procedure to a patient in the best way possible.

- Quality assurance includes scheduling, patient preparation, report generation, and quality control.

- **Quality control** deals with equipment and instrumentation.

- In diagnostic ultrasound, quality control consists of those procedures designed to monitor the performance of imaging apparatus.

- Quality control for digital ultrasound imagers is less demanding than that for analog imagers because the electronics are more stable.

- Quality control in diagnostic ultrasound consists of three principal areas: assessment of diagnostic accuracy, maintenance of imaging apparatus, and periodic equipment performance monitoring.

- Periodic equipment performance monitoring can involve the entire imaging team: the physician, the ultrasonographer, and the medical physicist.

- Performance monitoring is accomplished with the aid of test objects and phantoms.

- A test object is a geometric configuration designed to evaluate specific image or system parameters.

- The simplest test object is the Perspex plastic block.

- A 3-cm Perspex block can be used to monitor sensitivity, dynamic range, velocity (2680 m/s), and therefore distance calipers.

- Phantoms are anatomy-simulating devices.

$$1.74 \text{ cm perspex} = 1 \text{ cm soft tissue}$$

ten-point quality control program

Performance evaluation	Image rod group	Through surface
Sensitivity	B	D
Distance calibration	A, B	A, C, D
Caliper calibration	A, B	A, C, D
Registration	E	A/C and D/E
Dead zone	D	D
Axial resolution	E	D
Lateral resolution	C	A, C
Time-gain Compensation	A	D
Display characteristics	E	C, D

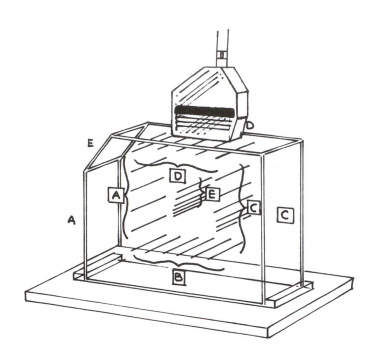

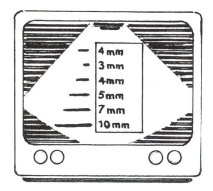

AIUM TEST OBJECT

- Of all available test objects, the AIUM (American Institute of Ultrasound in Medicine) device and its many modifications is the mostly widely employed.

- Essentially all test objects are constructed so that the velocity of sound in the test object is equal to that in soft tissue, 1540 m/s.

- The AIUM test object has five groups of rods identified as A to E.

- Group A consists of a vertical row—six rods spaced 20 mm apart.

- Group A is used to evaluate **depth calibration**, vertical linearity, and gain.

- Group B consists of a horizontal row of six rods spaced 20 mm apart at the bottom of the phantom.

- Group B rods are used to evaluate **sensitivity**, horizontal calibration, and horizontal linearity.

- Group C consists of seven rods spaced vertically at increments ranging from 3 to 25 mm.

- Group C rows are scanned from the side and used to evaluate **lateral resolution** and beam width.

- There are four rods in group D positioned at depths 2, 4, 6, and 8 mm, respectively from the top surface of the test object.

- Group D rods are used to evaluate the **dead zone** of the transducer.

- The dead zone is created by reverberation within the transducer and can worsen with physical damage or electronic faults.

- Group E consists of five rods positioned in the middle of the phantom and separated by 1, 2, 3, 4, and 5 mm.

- Group E rods are used to evaluate **axial resolution** and **registration**.

- A number of performance measurements can be completed with accuracy within just a few minutes' time.

SUAR TEST OBJECTS

- Sensitivity, uniformity, and axial resolution can be evaluated with an SUAR test object.

- SUAR test object is an acrylic block incorporating a water-filled wedge in a thermometer.

- The thermometer is required because ultrasound attenuation by the acrylic block increases with increasing temperature.

- The temperature must be maintained within a range of 20 to 22°C or a temperature correction factor applied.

- Sensitivity is evaluated by the position of controls—e.g., time-gain compensation, and amplifier gain—that will just permit visualization of the acrylic/air interface on the opposite side of the test object.

- Uniformity is evaluated by the image of the flat acrylic/air interface.

- The image should appear flat and of equal intensity across the field of view.

- Axial resolution is evaluated by imaging the fluid-filled wedge at the bottom of the test object.

- Each wedge surface is an acrylic fluid interface with a separation distance from 0 to 2.5 mm along its 100 mm length.

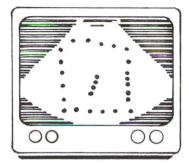
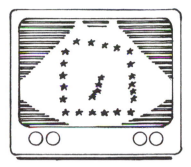
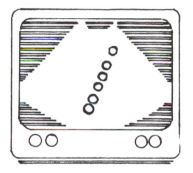
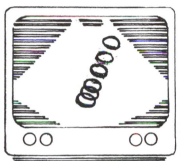

PHANTOMS

- There are tissue-mimicking phantoms of various designs to monitor image quality.

- Phantoms are available with simulated cysts or nodules.

- Phantoms are available with microscopic particles to simulate scattering and attenuation.

- Phantoms are available with various combinations of specular reflectors.

- Phantoms are available for Doppler flow evaluation.

- Phantoms are not as essential for a quality-control program as test objects are.

ROUTINE PERFORMANCE MEASUREMENTS

- Sensitivity measures the weakest echo that is detectable.

Routine Performance Monitoring

Task Measurement	Frequency	Recommended Performance
Distance	monthly	3 dB
Axial resolution	weekly	±2 %
Display	weekly	1 mm
Sensitivity	weekly	N/A
Caliper	monthly	± 2%
Registration	monthly	3 mm
Dead Zone	monthly	4 mm
Lateral Resolution	monthly	3 mm
TGC	monthly	N/A
Visual Inspection	monthly	N/A

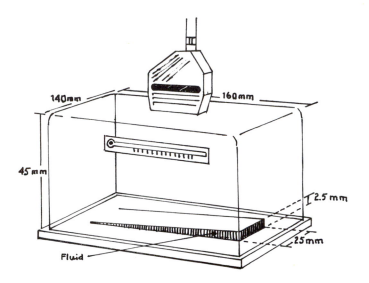

- Sensitivity is evaluated by recording the time-gain compensation (TGC) necessary to adjust image of an object at depth.

- Time or distance calibration is evaluated by imaging rods separated by 20 mm through the depth of the test object.

- When images of 20 mm separated rods do not measure 20 mm on hard copy, it indicates an inaccuracy in the speed of ultrasound or in the caliber calibration.

- When scanned from various angles, test objects should appear in the same position on the final image; if not, they are misregistered.

- There is a depth beyond the transducer phase where no echoes will be detected. This is the dead zone.

- The dead zone usually extends only 1 or 2 mm and is evaluated using group D rods of the AIUM phantom.

- Axial resolution is the ability of the ultrasound imager to image closely spaced reflectors along the axis of the ultrasound beam.

- Axial resolution is evaluated using closely spaced reflectors, such as the wedge of the SUAR test object or group E in the AIUM test object.

- Most ultrasound imagers will exhibit axial resolution of at least 1 mm.

- Lateral resolution is the ability to image reflecting objects in a plane perpendicular to the ultrasound beam axis.

- Lateral resolution is evaluated by imaging variously spaced reflectors positioned in a plane perpendicular to the ultrasound axis, such as group C rods in the AIUM phantom.

- Lateral resolution is usually in the 1 to 3 mm range.

- Time-gain compensation is a complex function of transducer frequency and test object depth.

- Each transducer should be evaluated for minimum TGC that will image reflectors at a depth, such as those in group A of the AIUM phantom.

- Evaluation of TGC setting is a frequent evaluation, to make sure that system electronics do not drift with time.

- As with any imaging apparatus, a visual inspection for frayed conductors or damaged transducers is appropriate.

Chapter 8 Review Questions

1. An error of distance measurement along the ultrasound beam axis occurs because of
   a. excessive noise.
   b. poor focusing.
   c. inaccurate focal depth.
   d. improper beam width.
   e. incorrect velocity calibration.

2. Which wire pattern is used to monitor axial resolution during a quality-control program?
   a. A
   b. B
   c. C
   d. D
   e. E

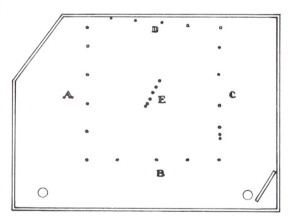

3. When processor QC is evaluated with a sensitometry film strip, which of the following is/are monitored?
   1. film speed
   2. film fog
   3. film contrast
   4. film resolution

   a. Only 1, 2, and 3 are correct.
   b. Only 1 and 3 are correct.
   c. Only 2 and 4 are correct.
   d. Only 4 is correct.
   e. All are correct.

4. **What is the name of the region near the skin when no useful echoes are obtained?**

   a. allowed zone
   b. B zone
   c. careful zone
   d. dead zone
   e. reflective zone

5. **Which wire pattern is used to monitor registration during a quality-control program?**

   a. A
   b. B
   c. C
   d. D
   e. E

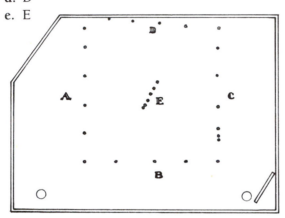

6. **The transducer should**

   1. be autoclaved when used during surgery.
   2. be autoclaved on a regular schedule.
   3. be autoclaved when a sterile field is required.
   4. not be autoclaved.

   a. Only 1, 2, and 3 are correct.
   b. Only 1 and 3 are correct.
   c. Only 2 and 4 are correct.
   d. Only 4 is correct.
   e. All are correct.

7. **In pulse echo (PE) imaging, inaccurate depth to echo is most likely due to**

   a. improper time-gain compensation (TGC).
   b. error in velocity calibration.
   c. incorrect attenuation coefficient.
   d. nonspecular reflection.
   e. too long a spatial pulse length (SPL).

8. **The best way to sterilize a transducer is to**

   a. autoclave it.
   b. use steam under pressure.
   c. irradiate it with gamma rays.
   d. follow manufacturer's instructions.
   e. use a commercial disinfectant.

9. Which wire pattern is used to monitor depth calibration during a quality-control program?

    a. A
    b. B
    c. C
    d. D
    e. E

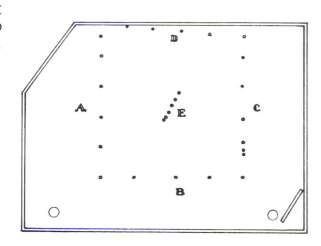

10. The American Institute of Ultrasound in Medicine (AIUM) performance-monitoring phantom can be used with what type of ultrasound imager?

    1. linear array
    2. phased array
    3. annular array
    4. simple B-mode

    a. Only 1, 2, and 3 are correct.
    b. Only 1 and 3 are correct.
    c. Only 2 and 4 are correct.
    d. Only 4 is correct.
    e. All are correct.

11. Which wire pattern is used to monitor lateral resolution during a quality-control program?

    a. A
    b. B
    c. C
    d. D
    e. E

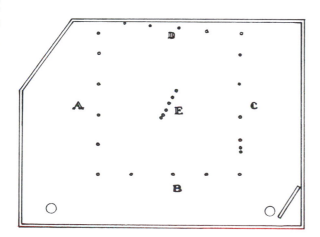

12. Which of the following detects a change in frequency?
    a. A-mode
    b. B-mode
    c. color-flow Doppler
    d. M-mode
    e. realtime

13. Which wire pattern is used to monitor dead zone during a quality-control program?
    a. A
    b. B
    c. C
    d. D
    e. E

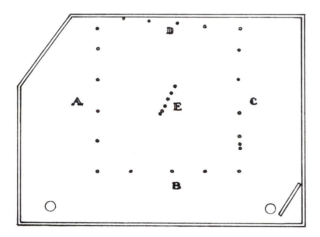

14. In order to map the beam-intensity profile, one should use a/the
    a. American Institute of Ultrasound in Medicine (AIUM) phantom.
    b. frequency analyzer.
    c. hydrophone.
    d. SUAR phantom.
    e. ultrasound dosimeter.

Biological Effects of Ultrasound

- When an imaging agent transfers energy to biological tissue, it occurs by the so-called **mechanism of action.**

- Diagnostic ultrasound interacts with tissue in two ways resulting in two effects—thermal effects and mechanical effects.

- In order to evaluate effects, one must have some knowledge of dosimetry, which is very difficult in diagnostic ultrasound.

- Ultrasound dosimetry is the study of intensity, power, pressure, pulse width, repetition rate, spatial dimensions, and exposure duration.

- Of the dosimetry measures, ultrasound intensity is perhaps the most difficult to evaluate yet the most important.

- Pulse echo (PE) ultrasound units produce SATA intensities of 5 to 20 mW/cm^2.

- Pulse echo ultrasound units produce SPTP intensities up to 10 W/cm^2.

- Doppler ultrasound units produce average intensities of 10 to 30 mW/cm^2.

- Mechanical effects have not been observed during diagnostic ultrasound.

- Ultrasonic physiotherapy systems operate at SATA intensities of 1 to 5 W/cm^2.

Power   watt (w)

intensity   milliwatt/cm^2 (mW/cm^2)

pressure   megapascals (MPa)

THERMAL EFFECTS

- Ultrasound causes tissue molecules to vibrate as waves of compression and rarefaction pass.

- Molecular vibration results in **tissue heating**.

- As ultrasound intensity and exposure time increase, tissue heating will increase.

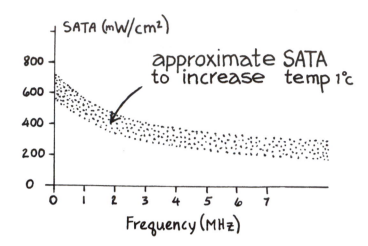

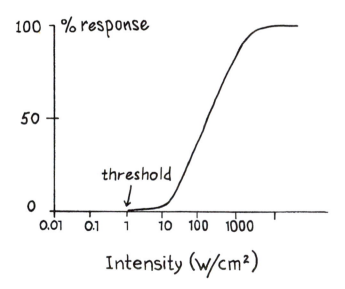

- A temperature rise of approximately 1°C is required to be physiologically measurable.

- Normal diurnal tissue variations can exceed 1°C; therefore, such temperature variation is considered totally safe.

- In the absence of the thermoregulatory ability of tissue, continuous ultrasonography at approximately 300 mW/cm^2 with a 2 MHz beam would be required for a 1°C rise in temperature.

- The body has two effective thermoregulatory properties—thermal **conduction** and thermal **convection**.

- Thermal conduction is transfer of heat from cell to cell by contact.

- Thermal convection is transfer of heat through blood flow.

- Highest temperature rise occurs in tissue in the region between the entrance skin and the focal region.

- Attenuation of the ultrasound beam results from absorption and scatter, but only absorption contributes to tissue heating.

- The higher the absorption coefficient (dB/cm/MHz) for a given tissue, the higher the rise in temperature.

- Soft tissue has low absorption, skin and cartilage have intermediate absorption, and both fetal and adult bone have high absorption.

- Amniotic fluid, blood, and urine absorb little ultrasound energy.

- Bone absorbs most ultrasound energy.

- Focusing an ultrasound beam increases temperature rise.

- For long-focus beams, the highest temperature rise will be nearer the surface.

- For short-focus beams, the highest temperature rise will be nearer the focal region.

- Scanned modes, such as B mode and color-flow Doppler, spread tissue heating more than unscanned modes, such as M mode and spectral Doppler.

- Continuous-mode ultrasound results in a higher temperature rise than pulsed mode.

- High-frequency ultrasound results in a higher temperature rise than low-frequency.

- The highest temperature rise in homogeneous soft tissue (abdominal exam) occurs just proximal to the focal region.

- The highest temperature rise in layered tissue (fluid-filled bladder to fetus) occurs in the fetus.

MECHANICAL EFFECTS

- There are two potential mechanical effects of ultrasound—**cavitation** and **microstreaming**.

- Cavitation occurs when dissolved gases become **microbubbles** during the rarefaction phase of the propagated ultrasound wave.

- Microbubbles can collapse, causing high temperature, membrane tear by shock wave, and free radical formation.

- Pulse echo ultrasound **cannot produce cavitation** because of the very short pulse lengths employed.

- Only sufficiently intense continuous-wave ultrasound can produce cavitation.

- Depending upon frequency, a resonance phenomenon can occur at a cavitation site, inducing microstreaming.

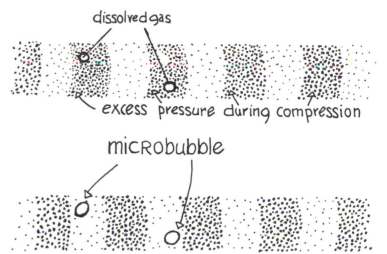

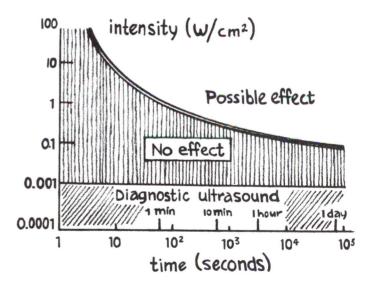

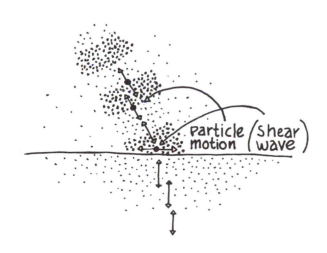

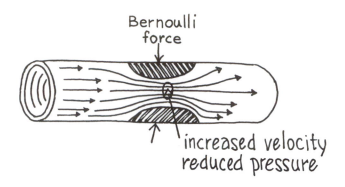

Bernoulli force

increased velocity reduced pressure

AIUM safety limits

$$I_{SPTA} < 100 \text{ m W/cm}^2$$

$$I_{SPTA} \times time < 50 \text{ J cm}^2$$
$$where \ 1s < time < 500s$$

USFDA recommended maximum intensity (mW/cm²)

Use	I_{SPTA}
cardiac	430
peripheral vessel	720
opthalmic	17
abdominal	94
fetal	94

- Microstreaming can result in high shear forces, which can possibly cause molecular breakage.

- Fluids (blood) passing through a constriction create the Bernoulli force, which tends to move the sides of the constriction to the center of flow.

- Ultrasound intensities less than 1000 mW/cm² cannot cause cavitation or microstreaming in any tissue.

- Mechanical effects are unimportant to diagnostic ultrasound.

CLINICAL SAFETY

- Thermal effects of diagnostic ultrasound are the only consideration.

- Benefit far outweighs presumed risk for diagnostic ultrasound.

- Practice the ALARA (As Low As Reasonably Achievable), principle.

- ALARA
  Select appropriate examination mode
  Select lowest appropriate frequency
  Select lowest appropriate pulse repetition frequency (PRF)
  Critically, select focal region
  Minimize examination time
  Optimize the examination, not the exposure time
  Minimize the American Institute of Ultrasound in Medicine (AIUM) indices: soft tissue thermal index (TIS), cranial bone thermal index (TIC), and bone thermal index (TIB)

Chapter 9 Review Questions

1. Which of the following labels the piezoelectric crystal?

   a. A
   b. B
   c. C
   d. D
   e. E

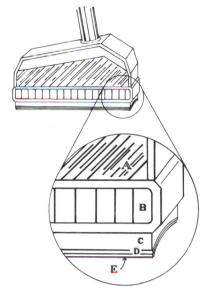

2. Which of the following is most closely related to biological effects?

   a. SATA
   b. SPPA
   c. SPTA
   d. SATP
   e. SPTA

3. The number of the thermal index is related to

   a. tissue temperature rise.
   b. acoustic intensity.
   c. time of exposure in seconds.
   d. time of exposure in minutes.
   e. intensity of exposure.

4. Which of the following labels the matching layer?

   a. A
   b. B
   c. C
   d. D
   e. E

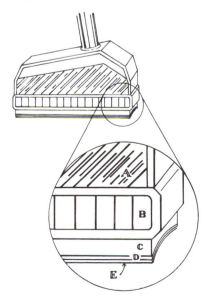

5. Which of the following is most closely related to possible biological effects?

   a. intensity in mW/cm^2
   b. power in dB
   c. Q value
   d. SPTP intensity
   e. TIB index

6. What are the two biological responses to ultrasound?

   a. absorption and attenuation
   b. attenuation and reflection
   c. direct and indirect
   d. ionization and excitation
   e. thermal and mechanical

7. If the ultrasound intensity is sufficiently high, what biological response could be produced?

   1. ionization
   2. excitation
   3. fusion
   4. cavitation

   a. Only 1, 2, and 3 are correct.
   b. Only 1 and 3 are correct.
   c. Only 2 and 4 are correct.
   d. Only 4 is correct.
   e. All are correct.

8. Which of the following labels the backing material?

   a. A
   b. B
   c. C
   d. D
   e. E

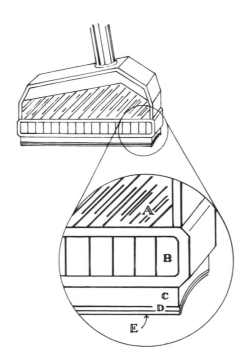

9. Cavitation is a biological response that results in

   a. atrophy.

   b. excitation.

   c. membrane sheer.

   d. microbubbles.

   e. necrosis.

10. Which of the following is a significant effect of diagnostic ultrasound?

   a. temperature decrease

   b. temperature increase

   c. membrane sheering

   d. atrophy

   e. nothing

11. Which of the following labels the transducer window?

   a. A

   b. B

   c. C

   d. D

   e. E

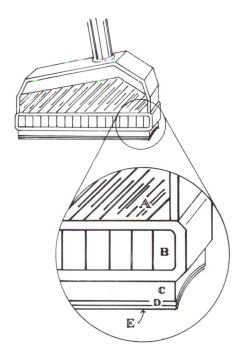

12. Absorption can be defined as

   a. bending of the ultrasound beam.

   b. scattering the ultrasound beam.

   c. converting the ultrasound energy into an electrical signal.

   d. converting the ultrasound energy into a mechanical disturbance.

   e. converting the ultrasound energy into heat.

13 The maximum Doppler shift frequency that is detectable equals

   a. one-half the center frequency.

   b. the center frequency.

   c. one-half the pulse repetition frequency (PRF).

   d. the pulse repetition frequency (PRF).

   e. twice the duty factor (DF).

14. Which of the following labels the damping material?
    a. A
    b. B
    c. C
    d. D
    e. E

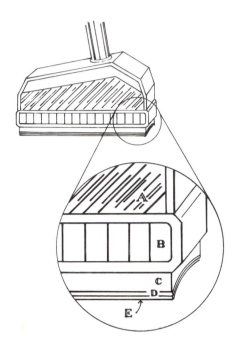

15. Which of the following is a biological response to ultrasound exposure?
    1. cavitation
    2. sheering
    3. heating
    4. conization

    a. Only 1, 2, and 3 are correct.
    b. Only 1 and 3 are correct.
    c. Only 2 and 4 are correct.
    d. Only 4 is correct.
    e. All are correct.

16. The number of the mechanical index is related to
    a. tissue temperature rise.
    b. acoustic intensity.
    c. sheer force.
    d. cavitation.
    e. intensity of exposure.

17. Reported biological responses of obstetric ultrasound include
    1. childhood malignancy.
    2. congenital abnormalities.
    3. neurologic deficit.
    4. cavitation.

    a. Only 1, 2, and 3 are correct.
    b. Only 1 and 3 are correct.
    c. Only 2 and 4 are correct.
    d. Only 4 is correct.
    e. None are correct.

18. Which of the following interactions is of most concern for causing biological effects?

    a. absorption
    b. dispersion
    c. diffraction
    d. reflection
    e. refraction

19. Epidemiologic studies of obstetrical ultrasound patients suggest the following biological responses.

    1. malignancy
    2. cataracts
    3. congenital abnormalities
    4. genetic effects

    a. Only 1, 2, and 3 are correct.
    b. Only 1 and 3 are correct.
    c. Only 2 and 4 are correct.
    d. Only 4 is correct.
    e. None are correct.

20. A diagnostic ultrasound beam passing through tissue can

    a. be totally attenuated.
    b. be totally transmitted.
    c. produce free radicals.
    d. produce ionization.
    e. elevate temperature.

Glossary

Abortion, complete   There are no retained products of conception and ultrasound scanning reveals a normal nonpregnant uterus containing a midline echo.

Abortion, incomplete   There are remaining products of conception in the uterus. The uterus appears bulky with no midline echo present and no evidence of a gestation sac.

Absorbed dose   The thermal energy imparted to matter by absorption of ultrasound per unit mass of irradiated tissue.

Absorbed dose rate   The time rate of increase of absorbed dose.

Absorber   Any material that absorbs ultrasound or reduces its intensity.

Absorption   Process by which ultrasound transfers energy to tissue by conversion of acoustic energy to heat. The cumulative effect of all forms of energy loss from an ultrasound pulse. Absorption contributes to attenuation.

Absorption coefficient   The fractional decrease in ultrasound intensity due to absorption in tissue.

Acoustic attenuation   Reduction of ultrasound intensity as a function of depth in tissue. Includes the effects of absorption, scattering, reflection, refraction and diffraction.

Acoustic coupling   A substance such as water, oil or gel that is placed on the skin to minimize the amount of air between the transducer and the skin, thereby achieving good acoustic transmission.

Acoustic energy   Mechanical energy transported by an ultrasound beam. Expressed as the product of acoustic power and time, or watt-second. 1 Ws = 1 J.

Acoustic enhancement   An artifact produced by over-amplification of ultrasound echoes lying behind fluid-filled or other poorly attenuating structures.

Acoustic holography   (See Holography).

Acoustic impedance   a. The ratio of ultrasound pressure at a tissue interface to its velocity at that interface. b. The product of ultrasound velocity (v) in a tissue of mass density (ρ). Expressed in rayls where 1 rayl = 1 $(kg/m^2 - s)$ (10^{-6}).

Acoustic impedance match   The condition of nearly equal acoustic impedances of contiguous media, avoiding reflection of ultrasound at the interface.

Acoustic impedance matching   The process whereby one or more layers of material with progressively lower acoustic impedance is placed on the front of an ultrasound transducer in an attempt to match the high impedance of the crystal to the low impedance of soft tissue.

Acoustic impedance mismatch   The condition of unequal acoustic impedances of contiguous media, causing reflection of ultrasound at the interface.

Acoustic intensity   Ultrasonic power transmitted per unit area. Expressed in mW/cm^2.

Acoustic lens   A refractive element such as a plastic or rubber lens placed in front of a flat crystal to focus the ultrasound beam.

Acoustic noise   Unwanted ultrasound signals caused mostly by multiple reflections or scattering of the ultrasound pulse.

Acoustic power   Acoustic energy per unit time (usually a temporal average is quoted). Expressed in W or J/s.

Acoustic pressure   The pressure inside a medium is alternately raised and lowered as a pulse of ultrasound passes through. The instantaneous value of the total pressure minus the ambient pressure. Expressed in megapascals, MPa.

Acoustic shadow   A manifestation of reduced ultrasound intensity in or returning from regions lying beyond an attenuating object. It is important to be able to distinguish between acoustic shadows and regions of low reflectivity.

Acoustic shadowing   An artifact produced by the loss of ultrasound intensity from structures lying behind an attenuating tissue or reflecting interface.

Acoustic streaming   An acoustically generated transport of fluid within that fluid or tissue.

Acoustic wave   A mechanical disturbance which travels through a medium such as tissue.

Acoustic waveform   (See Waveform).

Acoustic wavefront   The surface produced by wavelets in phase in a traveling wave.

Acoustic wavelength a. The distance between any adjacent points on a sinusoidal wave. b. The distance between any two similar adjacent points of an ultrasound wave. c. The distance traveled by the acoustic wavefront during one cycle. The wavelength of 1 MHz ultrasound in tissue is 1.54 mm.

Acoustic window An area of a patient, which is free from bone or gas, through which ultrasound can be passed to study deeper structures.

Acoustics a. The science of sound, including its production, transmission and effects. b. Containing, producing, arising from, actuated by, related to or associated with, subsonic, sound or ultrasound. May be replaced by the equivalent term "sonic" or when appropriate, the more specific "ultrasound".

Acute Something that begins suddenly and runs a short but rather severe course.

Adiabatic bulk modulus (K) The elastic modulus associated with the volume elasticity of fluid media when heat is not exchanged. The reciprocal of the adiabatic compressibility (β). $K = 1/\beta$.

Adnexa The structures occupying the para-uterine area, including the fallopian tube, broad ligament and ovary.

Agenesis Failure of development of an organ.

ALARA The principle requiring that ultrasound exposure be kept *As Low As Reasonably Achievable*; economic and social factors being taken into account.

Algorithm A computer-adapted mathematical calculation applied to the raw data during the process of image reconstruction.

Aliasing An artifact created by inadequate signal sampling.

Alpha-fetoprotein (AFP) One of the proteins present in amniotic fluid.

Alternating current Oscillation of electrons in both directions of a conductor.

American Association of Physicists in Medicine (AAPM) Scientific society of medical physicists.

American College of Medical Physicists (ACMP) Professional society of medical physicists.

American College of Radiology (ACR) Professional society of radiologists and medical physicists.

American Society of Radiologic Technologists (ASRT) Scientific and professional society of radiographers, radiotherapists, nuclear medicine technologists and ultrasonographers.

Amniocentesis Sampling of the amniotic fluid by inserting a needle into the uterus and withdrawing several ml of the fluid for analysis.

Amniotic fluid The fluid which surrounds the fetus *in utero*.

A-mode (amplitude-mode) A method of pulse echo display in which time is represented along the horizontal axis and amplitude is displayed along the vertical axis.

Amorphous tissue Tissue lacking echo-producing structures. These tissues include most cysts or other acoustically homogenous regions.

Ampere (A) The SI unit of electric charge. $1 A = 1 C/s$.

Amplitude a. The magnitude of the envelope or of the waveform of an ultrasound pulse. b. The maximum pressure or particle velocity during transmission of an ultrasound pulse.

Amplitude modulated waveform A waveform in which the carrier wave is modified in amplitude by a signal wave as a means of transmitting information.

Analog scan converter (See Scan converter).

Analog signal The continuous display of energy, intensity or ultrasound, as opposed to the discrete display of a digital signal.

Analog-to-digital converter (ADC) A computer which samples an analog signal at frequent regular intervals and converts it to a digital signal.

Anechoic The property of being echo-free or without echoes. A clear cyst is anechoic. (See Echogenic and Transonic).

Aneurysm An abnormal dilatation of an artery or cardiac chamber.

Aneurysm, false A collection of blood chambered outside of, but communicating with, the arterial lumen by a defect in the arterial wall.

Aneurysm, fusiform An aneurysm affecting a considerable length of an artery.

Angle of incidence a. The angle between the axis of an ultrasound beam at an interface and the perpendicular (normal) to the interface. b. That angle to the perpendicular made by the incident ultrasound beam, which is equal to the angle of reflection.

Angle of reflection The angle of the perpendicular made by the reflected ultrasound beam, which is equal to the angle of incidence.

Angstrom (Å) A unit of measure of wavelength. $1 \text{ Å} = 10^{-10}$ m.

Anhydramnios No amniotic fluid present.

Anisotropic Having different intensity in different directions.

Annotation Text added to images to provide descriptions or labeling.

Anteverted uterus The normal position of the uterus with the fundus pointing toward the anterior abdominal wall.

Arc scan An imaging technique in which the transducer is swept through an arc with its beam directed toward a fixed point.

Archival storage Secondary or permanent storage of digital images—usually magnetic tapes, magnetic disks or optical disks—and film images.

Array An arrangement of two or more transducer elements. The array may be a linear array or may be formed in other patterns such as hexagonal, annular or circular.

Array, annular   A circular transducer crystal that has been subdivided into several concentric rings each of which is energized separately.

Array, curvilinear   A type of realtime scanner in which a straight linear-array probe is bent into a curve to produce a sector form of image, thereby increasing the field of view with depth.

Array, linear   A type of realtime scanner consisting of a row of up to 600 small transducers side by side which are energized sequentially or segmentally.

Array, phased   A type of multielement realtime scanner where the ultrasound beam is electronically steered through a sector. A transducer configuration, which consists of multielements that can be excited independently. By proper phasing of the elements, a wavefront of the desired configuration can be synthesized. Phased arrays are utilized for electronic beam steering and focusing.

Array processor   That part of the computer that handles the raw data and performs the mathematical calculations necessary to reconstruct a digital image. Usually fixed, fast but inflexible.

Artifact   **a.** A pattern in an ultrasound image which is not a true representation of the anatomy under investigation. **b.** An apparent echo for which distance, direction or amplitude do not correspond to real tissue.

A-scan   A misnomer for A-mode. The procedure of scanning while viewing the A-mode display.

Atresia   Congenital obstruction of a hollow structure, commonly the small bowel or bile duct.

Attenuation   Reduction of ultrasound intensity when passing through tissue due to diffraction, absorption, scattering, reflection or any other process which redirects the echo away from the transducer. (See Acoustic attenuation).

Attenuation coefficient   Numerical expression of the decrease in intensity with distance in tissue. Expressed in dB/cm.

Attenuation compensation   Electronic compensation for attenuation due to losses and geometrical divergence of ultrasound; crafted to produce equal echoes from a reflector independent of depth. [See Time gain compensation (TGC)].

Attenuator   A device which reduces ultrasound intensity by a specified amount, e.g., in 10 dB steps.

Axial resolution   The minimum separation of reflectors along the ultrasound beam axis that can be separately distinguished.

Axial resolution   The minimum separation of reflectors along the direction of the ultrasound beam that can be separately distinguished on the display. (Same as depth resolution, longitudinal resolution and range resolution).

Azimuthal resolution   (See Lateral resolution).

Backscattered energy   The portion of the incident ultrasound beam reflected from a rough interface (compared to the wavelength) back toward the source; distinguished from specular reflection where the reflector dimension may be large compared to wavelength.

Baker's cyst   A cyst posterior to and communicating with the knee, filled with synovial fluid.

Bandwidth   The range of frequencies contained in an ultrasound pulse or echo.

Barium titanate (BaTiO$_3$)   A material belonging to a class of ferroelectric ceramics from which piezoelectric transducers are fabricated.

Beam   The acoustic ultrasound field produced by a transducer.

Beam axis   A straight line joining the points of maximum ultrasound intensity, at increasing distances from the transducer through the near field and into the far field.

Beam cross-sectional area   The area in a plane perpendicular to the beam axis that contains the ultrasound beam.

Beam divergence   The full angle of beam spread in a plane through the beam axis.

Beam uniformity ratio (BUR)   The ratio of the spatial peak-temporal average intensity (SPTA) to the spatial average-temporal average intensity (SATA) where both quantities are measured in a plane perpendicular to the beam axis.

Beam width   The width of the ultrasound beam in a plane perpendicular to the beam axis at a particular depth.

Bernoulli equation   An equation for determining the pressure drop in fluid passing through a narrow orifice. In cardiology a simplified form can be used for accurate prediction of the pressure drop across the cardiac valves.

Biliary sludge   A misnomer for the microcrystals which precipitate out within the gallbladder, leading to echoes in the most dependent part of the lumen. More correctly called *echogenic bile*.

Bioeffects   Change in the structure or function of tissues as a result of energy deposition.

Biparietal diameter (BPD)   The maximum distance between the fetal parietal eminences. An indicator of fetal age.

Bistable   A method of displaying B-mode information as black and white. No longer in use.

Bit   An abbreviation for binary digit. This is the numerical form in which computers and digital scan converters store information.

B-mode (Brightness-mode)   A method of ultrasound image display in which the intensity of the echo is represented by brightness and its location displayed in the x-y plane is determined by the position of the transducer and the transit time of the ultrasound pulse.

Breech A breech presentation occurs when the fetus has its buttocks adjacent to the internal os of the uterus.

Brightness-mode (See B-mode).

B-scan (See B-mode).

Bulk modulus (See Adiabatic bulk modulus).

Calibration The comparison of a laboratory source or instrument in daily use with a standard source or instrument to improve accuracy.

Calibration velocity The velocity of sound assumed during the calibration of an ultrasound imager, usually 1540 m/s.

Calipers Electronic cursors generated on a display that can be manipulated to coincide with echoes of interest for distance measurement.

Carcinogenesis Causing cancer.

Cardiomyopathy Disease of the heart muscle assumed to be caused by some agent other than coronary arterial disease.

Cathode ray tube (CRT) a. An electron beam tube designed for two-dimensional display of signals. b. A TV picture tube.

Cavernous hemangioma (See Hemangioma, cavernous).

Cavitation A phenomenon caused by high intensity ultrasound in tissue resulting in bubbles or cavities containing gas or vapor.

Cell The basic unit of all living matter.

Cell division Process whereby one cell divides to form two or more cells.

Cell membrane Structure encasing and surrounding the cell.

Cell metabolism Biochemical reactions necessary for cellular function, growth and reproduction.

Center for Devices and Radiological Health (CDRH) U.S. agency responsible for electronic radiation control program.

Center frequency The frequency determined by $(f_1 + f_2) / 2$, where f_1 and f_2 are the frequencies used to define bandwidth. Generally, the frequency at which the ultrasound amplitude is a maximum.

Cephalic presentation A cephalic presentation occurs when the fetus is lying longitudinally with its head in the lower part of the uterus.

Cholangiocarcinoma Malignant primary neoplasm of the biliary epithelium.

Cholecystitis Inflammation of the gallbladder wall, often associated with gallstones.

Choledochal cyst Congenital cystic dilatation of the common bile duct or major intrahepatic ducts.

Choriocarcinoma Malignant neoplasm of the placenta.

Chorionic plate The fetal surface of the placenta which is often visualized as a bright line between the placenta and amniotic fluid or fetus.

Choroid plexus Spongy bodies within the lateral ventricles of the brain which produce the cerebrospinal fluid.

Chromatid One of the two duplicate portions of DNA that appear as an arm of a chromosome.

Chromosome aberrations Visible changes in chromosome structure.

Chromosome analysis One of the tests which may be performed on amniotic fluid.

Chromosomes Small, rod-shaped bodies that contain the genes.

Chronic Something that continues for a long time as in disease or radiation exposure.

Cine loop A generic term used in ultrasound to describe the storage of a series of ultrasound images, typically the last 32–64 frames that can be replayed rapidly.

Cirrhosis A term describing abnormal growth of fibrous tissue in an organ.

Clipping (See Limiting).

Coarse gain An operational control provided on some diagnostic ultrasound systems for gross adjustments of amplifier gain.

Coefficient of variation The standard deviation divided by the value measured. $\sqrt{x}/x$

Collimator An acoustic lens used to focus an ultrasound beam.

Color-Flow Imaging (CFI) Production of a color overlay on a 2D image in which the blood flow direction and velocity information determine the color and hue assigned to each pixel in the color image.

Compound A chemical combination of two or more elements combined in a fixed and definite proportion.

Compound scan A method of scanning which combines at least two basic scanning motions.

Compressibility Ease with which a material can be compressed. (See Adiabatic bulk modulus).

Conductor Material that allows heat or electric current to flow relatively easy.

Congenital abnormalities Defects existing at birth that are not inherited but, rather, acquired during development *in utero*.

Congenital dislocation of the hip (CDH) Congenital displacement of the femoral head out of the acetabulum.

Contact coupling Acoustic coupling using gel or liquid to exclude air from the space between the transducer and skin.

Continuous wave (CW) An ultrasound beam of constant amplitude which exists for a large number of cycles as opposed to pulse echo (PE) ultrasound.

Contrast resolution Ability to detect and display similar tissues, such as gray matter–white matter, liver–spleen.

Control chart   A graphical plot of quality control test results with respect to time or sequence of measurement along with control limits.

Control limits   The limits shown on a control chart beyond which performance is compromised and corrective action required.

Cordocentesis   Ultrasound guided needling of the umbilical cord for fetal blood sampling.

Coronal plane   An imaging plane parallel to the long axis of the body and across the body, side to side.

Corpus luteum   A glandular structure which develops from the post-ovulation ovarian follicle.

Coulomb (C)   SI unit of electric charge.

Coupling medium   (See Acoustic coupling).

Covalent bond   A chemical union between atoms by sharing of one or more pairs of electrons.

Cross-over   Process that occurs during meiosis when chromatids exchange chromosomal material.

Cross-sectional display   A display which presents echo data from a single plane within a tissue.

Crown-rump length (CRL)   The maximum length of the embryo/fetus from the top of the head to the buttocks. Measurements of CRL by ultrasound are a valuable indicator of gestational age from 6 to 12 weeks of pregnancy.

Crystal   A colloquial term for the piezoelectric element of the ultrasound transducer. Many piezoelectric elements are made of polycrystalline materials.

Cursor   Electronic pointer used to outline areas of interest on a digital image for analysis.

Curvilinear array   (See Array, curvilinear).

Cytoplasm   The protoplasm that exists outside of the cell's nucleus.

Damping   Any material or mechanism that removes mechanical motion

from the ultrasound transducer. Damping is used to improve axial resolution.

Dead time   a. The time interval between the end of an emitted ultrasound pulse and the arrival of the first echo. b. The time between emitted ultrasound pulses.

Decibel (dB)   a. A unit used for expressing the ratio of two like quantities, such as electrical signal amplitude or ultrasound energy. b. Ten times the logarithm to the base ten of the ratio of two intensities, such as transmitted I_T and reflected I_R ultrasound $(dB = 10 \log \frac{I_R}{I_T})$.

Delay   A control to move the starting point of the TGC curve, normally only used when scanning through a water bath or full bladder.

Demodulator   a. An electronic circuit that removes the carrier frequency from a radio frequency signal. b. Ultrasound imagers use this circuit to remove the ultrasound frequency leaving the pulse echo envelope.

Densitometer   An instrument that measures the optical density of exposed film.

Deoxyribonucleic acid (DNA)   Molecule that carries the genetic information necessary for cell replication.

Depth gain compensation   (See Time gain compensation).

Depth of focus   The distance along the beam axis for a focussed transducer where the beam cross-sectional area is minimal. (See Focal zone).

Depth resolution   (See Axial resolution).

Deterministic effects   The severity of the biological response increases with increasing exposure. A dose threshold usually exists.

Dicentric chromosomes   Chromosomes having two centromeres.

Diffraction   The scattering of light or ultrasound when passing through a small aperture.

Diffuse reflection   Reflection that occurs at a tissue interface when surface roughness is smaller than or comparable to ultrasound wavelength. Reflection is over a wide range of angles, as opposed to specular reflection.

Diffusion   The motion of gas or liquid particles from an area of relatively high concentration to an area of lower concentration.

Digital scan converter   (See Scan converter).

Direct current   Flow of electrons in only one direction in a conductor.

Display format   The matter in which the ultrasound image is presented (e.g., A-mode, B-mode, etc).

Diverticulum   Congenital or acquired abnormal pouch or cul-de-sac extending from a hollow organ.

Dominant mutation   A genetic mutation that will probably be expressed in offspring.

Doppler angle   The angle between the axis of the Doppler ultrasound beam and the axis of the blood vessel under examination. This angle has to be measured to enable blood flow velocity to be computed.

Doppler effect   A shift in observed frequency caused by relative motion among source and/or receiver.

Doppler shift frequency   The difference between the frequencies of the transmitted pulse and the echo. It is proportional to the relative motion between the transducer and the reflector.

Doppler ultrasound   Application of the Doppler effect in ultrasound to detect wall movement, as in cardiac imaging or blood flow, as in vascular imaging.

Doppler, continuous wave   Detection of moving targets by the Doppler effect using a continuously transmitting transducer and a separate receiving transducer.

Doppler, pulsed A method of obtaining both velocity and depth information by detection of the Doppler shift frequency of pulse echoes.

Dosimetry The quantitative determination of spatial and temporal energy distributions and energy interaction with tissue.

Duplex scanning (See Scanning, duplex).

Duty cycle a. Ratio of "on time" to total exposure time during pulse echo ultrasound imaging. b. Ratio of the pulse duration to the pulse repetition time.

Duty factor The product of the ultrasound pulse duration and the pulse repetition rate.

Dynamic focusing A method of changing the focal zone of a transducer to produce multiple focal zones from a single transducer. The change of focusing using phase control of transmitted pulses. The use of multiple elements within a transducer to produce a curved wavefront, the shape of which can be changed to bring the beam to focus at different depths.

Dynamic imaging Imaging of an object in motion, a technique which is usually referred to as imaging in realtime.

Dynamic range a. The ratio in decibels of the maximum input signal which can be identified above noise. b. The ratio in decibels of the maximum input signal that can be displayed without reaching saturation to the smallest input signal that can be identified visually above noise. Expressed in dB.

Dysplasia Abnormal development of tissue.

Echo Ultrasound signal received from reflection at a tissue interface.

Echo ranging A technique for measuring distance in tissue by measuring the transit time for the ultrasound to travel from the transducer to the tissue interface and return.

Echocardiogram An echogram of the heart, most frequently an M-mode display.

Echocardiograph An instrument used to record an echocardiogram.

Echocardiography Examination of the heart by diagnostic ultrasound, using imaging, M-mode, color and spectral Doppler.

Echoencephalography Examination of the brain by diagnostic ultrasound, principally by using A-mode.

Echogenic Tissue that produces echoes in contrast to tissue which is free of echo-producing properties, not to be confused with highly reflective. (See Anechoic and Transonic).

Echogenic bile Bile which produces echoes as a result of hyperconcentration and the formation of microcrystals.

Echolucent A misnomer for anechoic and/or transonic.

Echoophthalmography An examination of the eye and orbit by diagnostic ultrasound.

Ectasia Abnormal dilatation of a tube or vessel.

Ectopic kidney A kidney which is situated other than in the renal fossa.

Ectopic pregnancy A pregnancy that becomes implanted outside the uterine cavity, usually in a fallopian tube.

Elastic modulus The ratio of stress to strain for any small disturbance from equilibrium. (See Adiabatic bulk modulus).

Elasticity The process, whereby tissue tends to restore itself when distorted to its undistorted configuration. (See Elastic modulus).

Electromotive force Electric potential. Expressed in volts (V).

Element Atoms having the same atomic number and same chemical properties. A substance that cannot be broken down further without changing its chemical properties.

Emaciation The state of being extremely thin.

Embryo The developing human from conception through approximately eight weeks (ten weeks from last menstrual period, LMP).

Embryo/fetus The developing human from conception until birth.

Embryological effects Damage that occurs as a result of toxic exposure of an organism during its embryonic stage of development.

Endometriosis The presence of secretory endometrioid tissue in an abnormal site.

Endoprobe An ultrasound imaging transducer designed for placement in a body cavity.

Energy Ability to do work. Expressed in joule (J).

Energy per pulse The ratio of the average acoustic power to the pulse repetition rate, measured in joule (J).

Envelope A continuous curve connecting the peaks of the successive cycles of the pulse echo (PE) waveform.

Epigastrium Middle part of the upper abdomen.

Epithelial tissue Tissue that covers the body and organs.

Error The difference between the measured value and the true value of a parameter or quantity.

Erythroblasts Red blood stem cells.

Erythrocytes Red blood cells.

Exposure time The total time the ultrasound transducer is delivering ultrasonic energy to the patient. In a pulse waveform this includes time between pulses.

Extremity Hand, elbow, arm below the elbow, foot, knee or leg below the knee.

False aneurysm (See Aneurysm, false).

False echoes (See Artifact).

Far field   The region of the ultrasound beam in which the acoustic energy along the beam axis diverges as though coming from a point source located near the transducer.

Fats   Compounds composed of carbon, hydrogen and oxygen with the ratio of hydrogen-to-oxygen being very much greater than 2-to-1.

Ferroelectricity   The dielectric phenomenon, analogous to ferromagnetism, by which a material spontaneously acquires piezoelectric properties through polarization.

Fetal ascites   Fluid in the fetal abdomen, usually occurring as a result of fetal cardiac failure.

Fetal blood sampling   (See Cordocentesis).

Fetus   The developing human from approximately the ninth week of pregnancy until birth (from ten weeks after the LMP until delivery).

Fibroid   A common benign tumor of the uterine muscle, more often multiple than single.

Focal area   The area of a surface in the focal zone perpendicular to the beam axis.

Focal length   The distance along the beam axis from a focusing ultrasound transducer to the depth of minimum focal area, the focal zone.

Focal surface   (See Focal area).

Focal zone   The narrower portion of the ultrasound beam produced by a focused transducer where there is best lateral resolution.

Focusing transducer   An ultrasound transducer assembly capable of fixed or dynamic focusing.

Focusing, dynamic   (See Dynamic focusing).

Focusing, fixed   Focusing of the ultrasound beam, usually with acoustic lenses, which cannot be altered.

Follicle   A normal cyst found in an ovary, which contains the developing ovum.

Force   That which changes the motion of an object. A push or pull. Expressed in Newtons (N).

Fractional bandwidth   The bandwidth divided by the center frequency.

Frame averaging   Reduction of noise in an image by adding together consecutive images. The signal is additive and the noise reduced by the square root of the number of frames averaged.

Frame freezer   A technique which allows the production of still frames from a realtime sequence.

Frame rate   The number of images per second.

Frame rate   The rate at which images are refreshed on the display of a realtime imager.

Fraunhofer zone   (See Far field).

Free radicals   Very reactive chemical molecules with unpaired electrons in the valence shell. Can be produced by ionizing radiation and ultrasound.

Frequency   Number of cycles or wavelengths of a simple harmonic motion per unit time. Expressed in Hertz (Hz). 1 Hz = 1 cycle/s.

Fresnel zone   (See Near field).

Gain   The ratio of the output to input of an amplifying system. Expressed in decibels (dB).

Gate   A device that can be switched electronically to control the transmission of a signal; for example, a range gate is designed to accept signals only from a specific frequency range. ECG triggered gate is designed to pass signals from a specified portion of the cardiac cycle.

Genes   The basic units of heredity.

Genetic effect   An effect in a descendant resulting from the modification of genetic material in a parent.

Germ cells   Reproductive cells.

Gestation sac   A fluid-filled structure containing the embryo/fetus.

Gigahertz   1000 megahertz. 10^9 Hz.

Glomerulonephritis   Inflammation of the kidney characterized primarily by changes in the glomeruli.

Grating lobe   Small side lobes of ultrasound energy emanating from the individual elements of a multi-element probe.

Gray scale   A term describing the property of an image display in which intensity is presented as variations in the brightness.

Hamartoma (angiomyolipoma)   A congenital malformation resembling a tumor but composed of multiple tissues which would not normally be present at the site, e.g., muscle, fat and cartilage in a kidney.

Hard copy   A permanent image on film or paper, as opposed to an image on a CRT, disk or magnetic tape.

Harmonic   A whole number multiple of the fundamental frequency; for example, the second harmonic of a 1 MHz wave is at 2 MHz. (Subharmonics also are possible; e.g., at ½, ⅓, etc. of the fundamental frequency).

Health physics   The science concerned with recognition, evaluation and control of radiation hazards.

Hemangioma, capillary   A congenital malformation of capillary blood vessels, which may be seen in the liver or kidney as a small, clearly defined highly reflective mass.

Hemangioma, cavernous   A congenital malformation of large blood vessels which may appear as a multicystic structure.

Hepatic adenoma   A rare benign neoplastic disorder of the liver which may be related to oral contraceptive consumption.

Hepatitis   Inflammation of the liver, usually caused by viral infection.

Hepatoma   A malignant primary tumor of the liver.

Hepatomegaly   Enlargement of the liver.

Hertz (Hz) Unit of frequency. Number of oscillations each second of a simple harmonic motion. Cycles per second.

Heterogeneous A term used to describe a structure or medium which has an uneven texture.

High pass filter An electronic circuit for selectively removing low frequency Doppler signals.

Highly differentiated cells Mature or more specialized cells.

Holography Three-dimensional imaging where tissue is uniformly irradiated with ultrasound and the reflected waves are sampled over a large area and summed with a reference wave, resulting in an interference pattern.

Homeostatis a. A state of equilibrium among tissue and organs. b. The ability of the body to return to normal function despite infection and environmental changes.

Homogeneous A term used to describe a structure or medium which has a uniform texture.

Hormones Proteins manufactured by various endocrine glands and carried by the blood to regulate body functions, such as, growth and development.

Hydrocalycosis Abnormal dilatation of the calyces of the kidney.

Hydrocephalus Abnormal dilatation of the intracerebral ventricles.

Hydrocephaly Abnormal fluid in the brain.

Hydronephrosis Abnormal dilatation of the renal collecting system.

Hydrosalpinx Abnormal dilatation of the fallopian tube.

Hyperechoic Producing echoes of higher amplitude than normal for the surrounding tissue.

Hypertrophic obstructive cardiomyopathy (HOCM) A disease of the heart muscle primarily affecting the upper portion of the ventricular septum which becomes thickened and obstructs the outflow of the left ventricle.

Hypoechoic Producing echoes of lower amplitude than normal for the surrounding tissue.

Image speckle A fine "snow storm" appearance seen in ultrasound images as a result of interference between the echoes arising from multiple different reflectors.

Immersion coupling A method of coupling an ultrasonic transducer to an object by placing both in a bath of the coupling medium.

Impedance (See Acoustic impedance).

Impedance ratio The ratio Z_2/Z_1, where Z_1 and Z_2 are the specific acoustic impedance of two contiguous tissues.

In vitro fertilization (IVF) A method of assisted conception whereby the ova are harvested from the mother, fertilized outside the body and the zygote or embryo inserted into the mother's uterine cavity.

Index of refraction The numerical value describing the bending of an ultrasound wave when passing from one tissue to another.

Inertia Property of matter that resists its change in motion or rest.

Insonation Application of sound to an object.

Insulator Material that inhibits the flow of electrons in a conductor or heat transfer.

Intensity A quantity related to acoustic power transmitted in a specified direction through a unit area normal to this direction. Expressed in mW/cm^2. (See Spatial average intensity, Temporal average intensity).

Intensity modulation Modification of the luminance of a display to represent information such as echo amplitude.

Interface The surface forming the boundary between two tissues having different acoustic impedance.

Interference The phenomenon in which two or more waves add (constructive) or cancel (destructive) according to their frequencies, amplitudes and phases.

Internal os The internal opening of the cervix.

International System of Units (SI) One standard system of units based on the meter, kilogram and second adopted by all countries and used in all branches of science.

Interphase The period of cell growth that occurs between cell divisions.

Interphase death Death of a cell before it attempts division.

Interpolation Calculation of a missing value from adjacent values in a numerical matrix or graph.

Intussusception Invagination of the bowel into itself, usually giving rise to obstruction and a palpable mass.

Ion An atom that has too many or too few electrons, causing it to have electric charge and to be chemically active. A free electron.

Ion pair Two oppositely charged particles.

Ionization Removal of an electron from an atom.

Ionize To remove an electron from an atom.

Ions Negatively and positively charged particles.

Isotropic Equal intensity in all directions. Having the same properties in all directions.

Isotropic scattering Scattering with equal energy distribution in all directions.

IUCD Intra-uterine contraceptive device.

IUD Intra-uterine death.

IUGR Intra-uterine growth retardation.

Joule (J) A unit of energy. The work done when a force of 1 Newton acts on an object along a distance of 1 meter.

Kilogram (kg) 1000 grams.

Kilohertz 1000 hertz. (See Hertz).

Kinetic energy Energy of motion.

Laminar flow Uniform and stable flow within a blood vessel in which the blood flows in concentric layers or streamlines, the flow within each layer being uniform in velocity. The highest flow velocity is in the center of the vessel and the velocity progressively falls towards the walls.

Laser Acronym from Light Amplification from Stimulated Emission of Radiation.

Lateral resolution The minimum separation of reflectors that can be imaged in a plane perpendicular to the ultrasound beam axis.

Lead metaniobate A ferroelectric ceramic used in transducers, $PbNiO_3$.

Lead zirconate titanate A ferroelectric ceramic used in transducers, $PbZrTiO_3$.

Leukemia A neoplastic overproduction of white blood cells.

Leukemogenesis The origin or production of leukemia.

Leukocytes White blood cells.

Limiting A technique that does not permit a voltage level to exceed a specified value.

Linear amplifier An amplifier for which the output is linearly proportional to the input.

Linear scan The motion of a transducer at constant speed along a straight line at right angles to the beam.

Linear-array (See Array, linear).

Lipids Water-insoluble organic macromolecules that store energy for the body consisting only of carbon, hydrogen and oxygen.

Liquid coupling (See Acoustic coupling).

Logarithmic amplifier An amplifier in which the output is proportional to the logarithm of the input.

Longitudinal a. Parallel with the beam axis. b. Parallel with the long axis of the body.

Longitudinal image plane (See Coronal or sagittal plane).

Longitudinal resolution (See Axial resolution).

Longitudinal wave Wave motion for which the particle displacement in the medium is in the direction of the wave and is perpendicular to the wavefront, (e.g., diagnostic ultrasound).

Lymphocele An abnormal collection of lymphatic fluid commonly caused by collections of lymph after severance of a lymphatic duct.

Lymphocyte A white blood cell that plays an active role in producing immunity for the body by producing antibodies.

Macromolecule Large molecule built from smaller chemical structures.

Manifest illness Stage of acute sickness during which signs and symptoms are apparent.

Mass Quantity of matter. Expressed in kilogram (kg).

Matching layer (See Acoustic impedance matching).

Matrix Rows and columns of pixels displayed on a digital image.

Matter Anything that occupies space and has form or shape.

Mechanical sector scanner (See Scanner, mechanical sector).

Mega (M) A numerical prefix equal to 1,000,000. (10^6)

Megahertz (MHz) One million cycles per second (10^6 Hz). (See Hertz).

Megapascal (MPa) A unit of pressure, 1 MPa = 10 atmospheres.

Meiosis The process of germ cell division which reduces the chromosomes in each daughter cell to half the number of chromosomes in the parent cell.

Metaphase That phase of cell division during which the chromosomes are microscopically visible.

Micro (μ) A numerical prefix equal to 10^{-6}.

Microcephaly Abnormally small size of the head.

Midline echo, fetal head This should be visible in the middle of the fetal head when the BPD is being measured.

Milli (m) A numerical prefix equal to 10^{-3}.

Milliwatt (mW) 1/1000 of a watt.

Mitosis The process of somatic cell division wherein a parent cell divides to form two daughter cells identical to the parent cell.

Mitotic delay The failure of a cell to start dividing on time.

M-mode (motion-mode) A method of ultrasound image display in which tissue depth is displayed on one axis and time is displayed along the second axis. M-mode is used frequently to display echocardiographic signals.

Moire pattern An artifact in a digital image caused by empty pixels resulting from attempts to display a diagonal line using a rectangular array of pixels.

Molecule A group of atoms of various elements held together by chemical forces. A molecule is the smallest unit of a compound that can exist by itself and retain all its chemical properties.

Monochromatic Having a single wavelength and therefore single frequency; usually referring to light.

Multicystic kidney A congenital malformation of the kidney associated with multiple cysts, little normal renal tissue and usually little renal function.

Multinodular goiter A benign condition of unknown cause associated with multiple nodules throughout the enlarged thyroid gland.

Multiplanar reformation Use of the original transverse images to produce images in another body plane.

Multiple matching layers (See Acoustic impedance, matching).

Mutations Changes in genes.

Myeloblasts White blood stem cells.

Myocarditis Inflammation of the cardiac muscle.

Nano (n) A numerical prefix equal to 10^{-9}.

Near field The region of an ultrasound beam lying between the transducer and the focal zone.

Near gain A means of varying the amplification of signals reflected from structures close to the transducer. These signals are larger than those received from more distant structures; therefore, they require less gain.

Necrosis Death of a portion of tissue.

Nephrocalcinosis Calcium deposition within the kidney.

Nephrosclerosis A form of kidney disease characterized by thickening in the walls of the renal vessels.

Neural tube defect (NTD) A congenital malformation of the brain or spinal canal.

Neutrophils A type of leukocyte that plays a role in fighting infection.

Newton (N) Unit of force in the SI system. 1 N = 0.23 lb.

Noise The grainy or uneven appearance of an image caused by a low signal or electronic interference.

Nonstochastic effects (See Deterministic effects).

Nonthermal effect A change in a medium or system due to energy absorption that is not directly associated with heat.

Nucleic acids Large, complex macromolecules involved with genes.

Nucleus a. The center of the living cell. A spherical mass of protoplasm containing the genetic material (DNA)

which is stored in its molecular structure. b. The curve of an atom, containing protons, neutrons and other subnuclear particles.

Oligohydramnios Too little amniotic fluid present.

Oogonium Female germ cell.

Orchitis Acute or chronic inflammation of the testis.

Organic compounds All carbon biochemical compounds.

Organogenesis Period of gestation from approximately the second to the eighth week after conception during which the nerve cells in the brain and spinal cord of the fetus develop and the fetus is most susceptible to congenital abnormalities.

Osteoporosis Decalcification of the bone.

Ovulation Release of an ovum by rupture of an ovarian follicle.

Pancreatitis Inflammation of the pancreas.

Papilloma A benign tumor on a stalk projecting from the surface of the skin or the endothelial lining of a hollow organ.

Parabolic flow (See Laminar flow).

Paradoxical movement Movement of a structure in the reverse direction to normal, e.g., upward movement of the diaphragm during inspiration.

Parenchyma All organs have a framework (stroma) of connective tissue that supports the specialized working tissue, parenchyma, that gives the organ its distinctive character.

Partial volume effect A structure such as a cyst that is smaller than the beam width appears to contain echoes, which are actually generated from surrounding tissue. Distortion of the signal intensity from a tissue structure because it extends partially into an adjacent slice thickness.

Particle velocity The velocity of a tissue molecule due to the passage of an acoustic wave.

Pelvic inflammatory disease (PID) Infection of the fallopian tubes, ovaries or the uterus.

Pelvimetry Ultrasonic or radiographic measurement of the female bony pelvis to insure that a fetal head will pass during delivery.

Penetration The depth an ultrasound beam passes into a tissue before its echoes become too weak to be detected.

Phantom A device which simulates some characteristics of tissue and allows measurement of ultrasound parameters or visualization of simulated anatomical features.

Phase Relating to the relative position of multiple ultrasound waves. When in phase, waves are aligned. When out of phase, wave position is random.

Phase contrast imaging A method of imaging the structure of tissues by sensing small variations in phase velocity.

Phased-array (See Array, phased).

Pico (P) A numerical prefix equal to 10^{-12}.

Piezoelectric effect The property exhibited by certain crystals of generating electrical potentials when mechanically stressed. Conversely, these crystals generate mechanical strains when electrically stressed.

Pixel A discrete picture element in a digital image.

Placenta previa A placenta which extends into the lower segment of the uterus.

Placental abruption Separation of the placenta from the uterine wall.

Placental grading A system for describing the ultrasound imaging characteristics of the placenta.

Placental infarction Death of an area of the placenta caused by obstruction to or thrombosis of the placental vessels.

Plane wave A propagating wavefront that approximates a plane; ideally, a wavefront at infinite distance from a point source but in most cases considered to be a wavefront in the far field.

Platelets Circular or oval disks found in the blood that initiate blood clotting and prevent hemorrhage.

Plug flow Uniform flow within a blood vessel in which there is the same velocity across the vessel profile.

Point mutation Genetic mutations in which the chromosome is not broken but the DNA within it is damaged by the breaking of a single chemical bond.

Polycystic infantile type Usually manifest at birth by enlargement of the kidneys which are highly reflective on ultrasound.

Polycystic liver disease A congenital familial disorder in which numerous varying sized cysts appear within the liver in adulthood.

Polycystic renal disease A congenital familial disorder of the kidneys whereby numerous cysts appear within the renal parenchyma, usually in adult life.

Polyhydramnios Too much amniotic fluid present.

Porencephalic cyst An acquired cystic lesion within the cerebral hemisphere but communicating with the ventricular system.

Portal hypertension Abnormal increase in the blood pressure within the portal venous system.

Posterior hypertension The vitreous-filled cavity posterior to the lens.

Postprocessing Changing the appearance of a digital image by manipulation of the raw data, e.g., smoothing, edge enhancement, zoom, etc.

Potential difference The difference in voltage between two points in a circuit.

Power Rate at which work is done. The rate of change of energy with time. Expressed in watts (W). 1 W = 1 J/s.

Pressure (See Acoustic pressure).

Prophase The phase of cell division during which the nucleus and the chromosomes enlarge and the DNA begins to take structural form.

Protein Amino acids that link together in various combinations and patterns.

Protocol A procedure to be used when performing a quality control measurement or standard imaging procedure.

Protoplasm The building material of all living things.

Pseudocyst A false cyst-like structure developing in tissues.

Pseudogestation sac A collection of fluid within the uterine cavity giving an appearance similar to that of a gestation sac.

Pseudokidney An ultrasound appearance similar to that of a normal kidney but usually produced by abnormal thickening of the bowel wall.

Pulsatility index A mathematical formula for assessing the pulsatility of Doppler blood flow waveforms. Peak to peak velocity or frequency ÷ mean velocity or frequency.

Pulse A brief burst of ultrasound, normally about 1 microsecond in duration.

Pulse average intensity (PA) The time-average of ultrasound intensity over the pulse length.

Pulse duration (PD) The time interval that an ultrasound pulse exists. This term is preferable to pulse length.

Pulse echo technique (See Echo ranging).

Pulse length (PL) The distance in tissue of an ultrasound pulse. Typically, 1–3 μm. (See Pulse duration).

Pulse repetition frequency (PRF) The rate at which ultrasound pulses are produced. Typically, in the range from 1 to 5 kHz. Also called pulse repetition rate. PRF = 1/PRP.

Pulse repetition period (PRP) The time interval between the same point on the waveform of two successive ultrasound pulses. The inverse of pulse repetition frequency. PRP = 1/PRF.

Pulse repetition rate (See Pulse repetition frequency).

Pulsed Doppler (See Doppler, pulsed).

Pyloric stenosis A condition of unknown cause occurring in infants and characterized by abnormal thickening of the pyloric muscle, giving rise to gastric outlet obstruction.

PZT (See Lead zirconate titanate).

Quality assurance All those planned and systematic actions necessary to provide adequate confidence that a facility, system or administrative component will perform safely and satisfactorily in service to the patient. Includes scheduling, preparation and promptness in the examination or treatment and reporting the results, and quality control.

Quality control Included within quality assurance, comprises all those actions necessary to control and verify the performance of equipment.

Quartz A piezoelectric crystal used in transducers.

Radicals Groups of atoms that remain together during a chemical change behaving almost like a single atom.

Radio frequency (RF) The frequency(ies) of the signals at the electrical terminals of the transducer; the frequency(ies) of signals from the transducer before detection.

Radiological Society of North America (RSNA) Scientific society of radiologists and medical physicists.

Radiologist A qualified physician who specializes in medical imaging using x-rays, radioactive material, ultrasound and MRI.

Radiology That branch of medicine dealing with the diagnostic and therapeutic applications of radiation.

Random errors Errors that vary in a nonreproducible way around the mean.

Range gate The time or distance during which echoes are accepted in a pulsed Doppler system.

Range resolution (See Axial resolution).

Rayleigh scattering Near isotropic scattering by a particle having dimensions much smaller than the wavelength of the incident acoustic radiation in accordance with the theory developed by Rayleigh.

Realtime (See Realtime display).

Realtime display A display for which the image is continuously renewed, keeping pace with changes in the object and in which storage or processing time does not delay appreciably the image presentation.

Realtime scanner (See Scanner, realtime).

Recessive mutation A genetic mutation that will probably not be expressed for a number of generations because both parents must possess the same mutation for expression.

Reconstruction Creating an image from data.

Reflected acoustic pulse . (See Echo).

Reflected wave (See Echo).

Reflection Reversal of the direction of an ultrasound beam when it encounters an extended interface with another tissue of different acoustic impedance.

Refraction The phenomenon of bending wavefronts and changing the direction of ultrasound as it passes from a medium of one acoustic velocity to a second medium of differing acoustic velocity.

Region of interest (ROI) An area of anatomy defined by the operator using a cursor on a reconstructed digital image.

Registration A quality of the display related to the accuracy of the position of tissue reflections; usually referring to the summation of images.

Rejection A technique to improve the apparent signal-to-noise ratio by eliminating low-amplitude signals from a display. (See Suppression).

Relaxation A class of processes in which acoustic energy is absorbed in a medium. Return of a disturbed tissue molecule to its original position following the passing of an ultrasound pulse.

Renal agenesis Failure of formation of a kidney.

Reproductive cells Male and female germ cells.

Resistance index (Pourcelot index) A simple mathematical formula for relaxing peak systole (PS) to end diastole (ED). $\frac{PS-ED}{PS}$

Resolution A measure of the ability of a system to image two closely spaced structures.

Retinal detachment Abnormal separation of the retina from the other layers of the eye.

Retroverted uterus A uterus which lies with the fundus pointing backwards towards the sacrum.

Reverberation The phenomenon of multiple reflections; usually between the transducer and a strong interface lying parallel to the transducer. Echoes are misplaced on the image, creating an artifact.

Ribonucleic acid (RNA) A type of nucleic acid that carries the genetic information from the DNA in the cell nucleus to the ribosomes located in the cytoplasm.

Rise time The time taken for an ultrasound pulse or echo amplitude to increase from its minimum to maximum peak value.

Rotating probe (See Scanner, mechanical sector).

Sagittal plane An imaging plane parallel to the long axis of the body and through the body, front and back.

Scalar Quantity or measurement that has only magnitude, as opposed to vector, which also has direction.

Scan The moving of an ultrasound beam to produce an image, for which the transducer and the display movements are synchronized in space and time.

Scan converter The device that converts signal data to an image. The type of scan converter in general use today is digital, where the image is stored in binary code in a solid state computer memory.

Scan repetition rate (See Frame rate).

Scan, sector (See Sector scan).

Scanner A device to produce an axial or transaxial sectional image.

Scanner a. A piece of equipment designed to produce an ultrasound image. Preferred terminology is imager. b. Sometimes used to describe the ultrasonographer.

Scanner, mechanical sector A realtime system in which the scanning is undertaken by oscillation or rotation of the transducer(s).

Scanner, realtime A device whose image is continuously renewed so that it keeps pace with the changes in the object being scanned and in which storage or processing time does not delay the image presentation.

Scanning, duplex The simultaneous acquisition of a 2D image and pulsed Doppler information.

Scanning, triplex Simultaneous 2D gray scale imaging, pulsed Doppler and color flow imaging.

Scattering The diffuse reflection, refraction or diffraction of ultrasound in many directions from irregular tissue surfaces or inhomogeneities to be changed in direction, frequency, phase or polarization.

Scattering angle The angle, θ, between the incident wave and final direction of a scattered wave in a particular observation.

Sector scan   A slice-of-pie image produced when the transmitted beam is rotated through an angle, the center of rotation being near or behind the surface of the transducer.

Sensitivity   The minimum signal that can be detected; usually, limited by the noise of the system.

Shear modulus   (See Elastic modulus).

Shear wave   Wave motion with particle movements perpendicular to the direction of travel. Shear waves are generated when a longitudinal wave impinges obliquely on soft tissue–bone interfaces and partially account for the heating of the periosteum and bone at this location.

Shock wave   A distorted and very brief ultrasound pulse in which the peak amplitude and rate of change of energy are greatly increased.

Side lobe   A diffraction phenomenon occurring at the edges of an ultrasound beam in which secondary, off-axis maxima occur in the near or far field or in the focal zone. Side lobes are more pronounced in array systems and are suppressed with electronic techniques such as shading. Side lobes tend to limit lateral resolution.

Signal   The information content of the variation in current or voltage in a receiver.

Signal-to-noise-ratio (SNR)   Sensitivity of a detector to recognize signal in the presence of background noise.

Sinusoidal   Simple harmonic motion. A sine wave.

Slice thickness   The effective thickness of tissue examined by ultrasound.

Somatic cells   All of the cells in the human body with the exception of the germ cells.

Sonar   Acronym from *SO*und *NA*vigation *R*anging.

Sonography   Any imaging method using sound and yielding a graphical representation of the tissue. This is a more inclusive term than ultrasonography.

Sonolucent   A misnomer for transonic or anechoic with low absorption.

Sound   Propagating vibrational energy within a medium. (See Acoustic energy).

Sound pressure amplitude   The deviation from the ambient value of the pressure in a medium due to the passing of an acoustic wave.

Spatial average intensity (SA)   The ultrasound intensity averaged over the ultrasound beam cross-sectional area. Generally, this parameter is used when specifying the intensity for continuous wave (CW) ultrasound.

Spatial average, pulse average intensity (SAPA)   The mean of the spatial average ultrasound intensity throughout the duration of the pulse.

Spatial average, temporal average intensity (SATA)   The mean of the spatial average ultrasound intensity over a time period which includes several pulses and the intervals between the pulses.

Spatial average, temporal average intensity (SATA)   The temporal average ultrasound intensity averaged over the beam cross-sectional area.

Spatial frequency   A method of expressing size. The number of cycles per unit distance for a periodic waveform. A measure of the changes of tissue attenuation characteristics. Abrupt changes in tissue (e.g., bone–lung interface) have high spatial frequency and gradual changes (e.g., liver–spleen) have a low spatial frequency. Expressed in line pairs per millimeter (1p/mm).

Spatial peak, pulse average intensity (SPPA)   The value of the pulse average intensity at the point in the ultrasound beam where the pulse average intensity is a maximum or is a local maximum within a specified region.

Spatial peak, temporal average intensity (SPTA)   The maximum intensity within an ultrasound beam - usually at the center of focal zone - averaged over time.

Spatial peak, temporal average intensity (SPTA)   The value of the temporal average ultrasound intensity at the point in the beam where the temporal average intensity is a maximum or is a local maximum within a specified region.

Spatial peak, temporal peak intensity (SPTP)   The maximum intensity within an ultrasound beam during the passage of the peak of the pulse.

Spatial peak, temporal peak intensity (SPTP)   The value of the temporal peak ultrasound intensity at the point in the ultrasound beam where the temporal peak intensity is a maximum or is a local maximum within a specified region.

Spatial resolution   The ability to image anatomical structures or small objects of high contrast.

Speckle   The granular appearance of an image due to a weak signal and electronic noise.

Spectral analysis   A method of analyzing a wavefront, such as ultrasound pulse, by providing the amplitude and phase as a function of frequency of its component waves.

Spectral analysis   A method of analyzing the frequency content of the Doppler signal and displaying it graphically.

Spectral broadening   Increase in the frequency bandwidth of a Doppler ultrasound signal caused by disturbances in blood flow around a stenosis.

Spectrum   Graphic representation of the range over which a quantity extends, e.g. frequency spectrum.

Specular reflection   Reflection from surfaces that are smooth compared to the wavelength of sound. In contrast to diffuse reflections from rough surfaces, specular reflection is highly directional. Mirror-like reflection.

Speed of sound The product of the frequency (f) and the wavelength (λ) in tissue. $v = f\lambda$. Expressed in m/s.

Spermatocele Abnormal cystic dilatation of the epididymis.

Spermatogonium The male germ cell.

Splenomegaly Enlargement of the spleen.

Spontaneous mutations Mutations in genes that occur at random and without a known cause. A natural mutation.

Standard A material or substance the properties of which are believed to be known with sufficient accuracy to permit its use to evaluate the same property of other materials.

Stem cells Immature or precursor cells.

Stochastic effects The probability or frequency of the biologic response is a function of exposure. Disease incidence increases proportionately with exposure and there is no dose threshold.

Streaming The production of non-physiological movement in tissue or cellular fluids during ultrasound exposure.

Superposition Imaging overlying tissues as in radiography.

Suppression The elimination of selected ultrasound signals; usually weak signals below a threshold level. (See Rejection).

Swept gain The gain of a pulse echo system is varied with time to compensate for the effects of attenuation. (See Time gain compensation).

Systematic errors Errors that are reproducible and tend to bias a result in one direction.

Temporal average intensity (TA) The time-average of ultrasound intensity at a point in tissue.

Temporal peak intensity (TP) The peak value of ultrasound intensity at the point in tissue considered.

Teratogenesis A process leading to the development of fetal abnormalities.

Test object A passive device which provides echoes and permits evaluation of one or more parameters of an ultrasound system but does not necessarily duplicate the acoustical properties of the human body. (See Phantom).

Testicular seminoma A primary malignant neoplasm of the testis.

Testicular teratoma A primary malignant neoplasm of the testis.

Tetralogy of Fallot A congenital abnormality of the heart that includes ventricular septal defect, overriding the aorta over the defect, pulmonary stenosis and an abnormal aortic arch.

Thermal energy Energy of molecular motion—heat.

Threshold dose The dose at which a response to an increasing intensity first occurs. Threshold dose is also that dose below which there is no biological response.

Thrombocytes (See Platelets).

Thymus gland An organ of the lymphatic system, located in the mediastinal cavity anterior to and above the heart.

Thyroid gland An endocrine gland located in the neck just below the larynx.

Time base The (real or virtual) trace on a display representing the time coordinate.

Time gain compensation (TGC) Increase in gain with time to compensate for loss in echo amplitude due to attenuation with depth.

Tissue equivalent material Material that exhibits one or more acoustic properties qualitatively and/or quantitatively similar to those of specific tissue.

TM and TP-mode (See M-mode).

Transceiver A transducer used for both transmission and reception of ultrasound.

Transducer A device capable of converting energy from one form to another. The device used in ultrasound to convert electrical energy to mechanical energy and vice versa.

Transducer assembly That portion of a diagnostic ultrasound imager which is designed to emit and/or receive ultrasound and which includes one or more transducers in a hand-held housing.

Transition zone That portion of the ultrasound beam having no distinct boundaries at the near field/far field interface. (See Focal zone).

Transonic Tissue that is relatively unattenuating. A distinction should be made between a transonic region and a shadowing region. (See Anechoic and Echogenic).

Transverse wave a. The type of waves present when ultrasound is conducted across the surface of water and along the surface of bone. The particles move at right angles to the direction of travel of the pulse. b. The particle or energy disturbance is at right angles to the propagation as with electromagnetic radiation. (See Shear wave).

Trimester The gestational period is divided into three stages of approximately three months each.

Triplex scanning (See Scanning, triplex).

Ultrasonic shadow (See Acoustic shadow).

Ultrasonic transducer (See Transducer).

Ultrasonogram Any image obtained using diagnostic ultrasound.

Ultrasound Acoustic radiation at frequencies above the range of human hearing, approximately 20 kHz.

Uncertainty The range of values within which the true value is estimated to lie.

Undifferentiated cells Immature or nonspecialized cells.

Ureterocele An abnormal dilatation of the lower intravesical portion of a ureter caused by congenital narrowing of the ureteric orifice.

Valence electrons Electrons in the outermost shell of an atom.

Vector Quantity or measurement that has magnitude and direction, as opposed to scalar.

Velocity The term *velocity* implies both direction and speed; the term *speed of sound* should be used where direction is not important. (See Speed of sound).

Visual acuity Ability to discriminate small image patterns.

Voltage Electric potential relative to ground potential. The volt (v) is the SI unit of electric potential and potential difference.

Vortex Swirling rotational blood flow similar to a whirlpool, usually occurring distal to a stenosis or vascular branch.

Voxel A *volume element*. Similar to a pixel in a 2D image but including the slice thickness.

Wall thump High-amplitude, low-frequency Doppler signals produced by the pulsatile movement of the walls of arteries.

Wall thump filter (See High pass filter).

Wave (See Acoustic wave).

Waveform The representation of an acoustical or electrical parameter as a function of time.

Wavefront A complex ultrasound pulse produced by the additive effect of multiple small pulses (wavelets) generated by the elements of a multielement array transducer.

Wavelength (See Acoustic wavelength).

Weight Force caused by the acceleration of gravity on a mass. Properly expressed in Newtons (N) but commonly expressed in pounds (lb). 1 lb = 4.4 N.

Window level The location on the digital image number scale where the levels of grays will be assigned. Regulates the optical density of the displayed image.

Window width Assigning a specific number of gray levels or digital image numbers to an image. Regulates the contrast of the displayed image.

Work Product of the force on an object and the distance over which the force acts. Expressed in joule (J). W = Fd.

Appropriate Textbooks

Bushberg JT, Seibert JA, Leidholdt EM Jr, Boone JM: **The Essential Physics of Medical Imaging.** Williams and Wilkins, Baltimore, MD, 1994.

Bushong SC, Archer BR: **Diagnostic Ultrasound–Physics, Biology and Instrumentation.** Mosby-Year Book, St. Louis, MO, 1991.

Fish P: **Physics and Instrumentation of Diagnostic Medical Ultrasound.** John Wiley & Sons, Chichester, 1990.

Hedrick WR, Hykes DL, Starchman DE: **Ultrasound Physics and Instrumentation–Practice Examinations.** Mosby-Year Book, St. Louis, MO, 1995.

Hedrick WR, Hykes DL, Starchmann DE: **Ultrasound Physics and Instrumentation**, 3rd ed. Mosby-Year Book, St. Louis, MO, 1995.

Huda W, Slone RM: **Review of Radiologic Physics.** Williams and Wilkins, Baltimore, MD,1995.

Kremkau FW: **Diagnostic Ultrasound-Principles, Instruments and Exercises**, 3rd ed. W.B. Saunders Company, Philadelphia, PA, 1989.

Kremkau FW: **Doppler Ultrasound–Principles and Instruments.** W.B. Saunders Company, Philadelphia, PA, 1990.

Kisslo J, Adams DB, Belkin RN: **Doppler Color Flow Imaging.** Churchill Livingstone, New York, NY, 1988.

Meire HB, Farrant P: **Basic Ultrasound.** John Wiley & Sons, Chichester, 1995.

Odwin CS, Dubinsky T, Fleischer AC: **Appleton & Lange's Review for the Ultrasonography Examination**, 2nd ed. Appleton & Lange, Norwalk, CT, 1993.

Smith H-J, Zagzebski JA: **Basic Doppler Physics.** Medical Physics Publishing, Madison, WI, 1991.

Sprawls P Jr: **Physical Principles of Medical Imaging.** Aspen Publishers, Gaithersburg, MD, 1993.

Zagzebski. JA: **Essentials of Ultrasound Physics.** Mosby, St. Louis, MO, 1996.

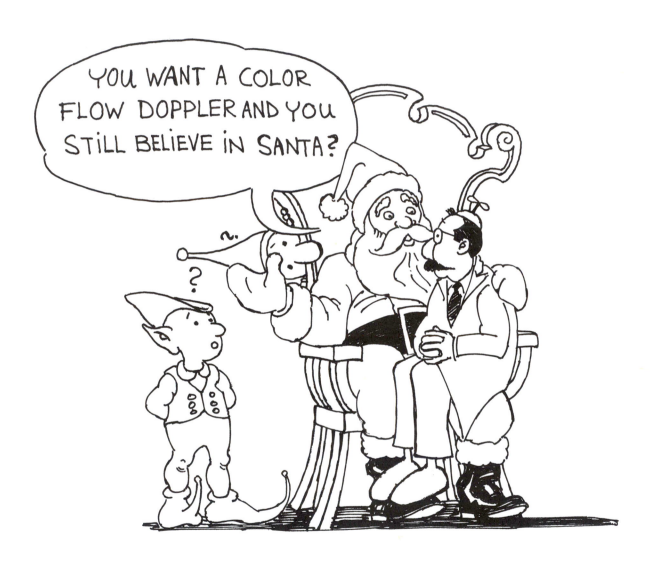

Answers

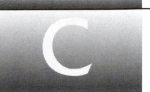

Chapter 1
1. c
2. b
3. b
4. c
5. d
6. d
7. c
8. a
9. c
10. e
11. c
12. d
13. b
14. a
15. b
16. e
17. b
18. d
19. c
20. d
21. c
22. d
23. a
24. a
25. b
26. d
27. d
28. e
29. d
30. e
31. c
32. b
33. c
34. a
35. d
36. a
37. e
38. d
39. e
40. a
41. e
42. b

43. d
44. a
45. d
46. d
47. d
48. b
49. a
50. e
51. e
52. a
53. a
54. b
55. c

Chapter 2
1. c
2. c
3. a
4. e
5. b
6. b
7. d
8. b
9. d
10. e
11. b
12. c
13. b
14. a
15. a
16. c
17. b
18. b
19. c
20. e
21. c
22. e
23. d
24. d
25. b
26. d
27. e
28. d

29. e
30. a
31. e
32. b
33. e
34. c
35. e
36. a
37. d
38. e
39. c
40. d
41. c
42. d
43. d
44. d
45. e
46. b
47. c
48. c
49. a
50. c
51. a
52. e
53. e
54. c
55. c
56. e
57. e
58. c
59. e
60. e
61. a
62. a
63. a
64. d
65. c
66. c
67. d
68. d
69. a
70. d
71. a

72. e
73. e
74. a
75. c

Chapter 3
1. d
2. d
3. d
4. e
5. c
6. c
7. d
8. e
9. c
10. e
11. a
12. a
13. e
14. a
15. c
16. c
17. c
18. d
19. a
20. d
21. e
22. b
23. c
24. a
25. b
26. d
27. a
28. c
29. b
30. c
31. d
32. e

Chapter 4
1. d
2. d
3. a

4. a
5. b
6. c
7. a
8. a
9. b
10. b
11. d
12. c
13. c
14. d
15. b
16. a
17. c
18. a
19. d
20. c
21. c
22. c
23. a
24. c
25. b
26. a
27. c
28. b
29. c
30. b
31. c
32. a
33. b
34. a
35. e
36. c
37. d
38. a
39. d
40. d
41. a
42. e
43. e
44. c
45. a
46. a
47. d
48. a
49. a
50. b
51. b
52. c
53. d
54. b
55. d
56. c
57. e
58. e
59. b

60. c
61. c
62. d
63. e
64. c
65. c
66. e
67. a
68. e
69. a
70. a
71. c
72. b
73. a
74. b

Chapter 5
1. b
2. e
3. c
4. c
5. d
6. c
7. e
8. e
9. b
10. b
11. b
12. a
13. c
14. c
15. a
16. b
17. b
18. c
19. a
20. d
21. c
22. b
23. b
24. c
25. d
26. d
27. b
28. c
29. d
30. b
31. b
32. b
33. e
34. a
35. e
36. b
37. d
38. d
39. c

40. e
41. a
42. b
43. d
44. e
45. d
46. c
47. e
48. a
49. c
50. b
51. e
52. d
53. e
54. c
55. e
56. a
57. b
58. a
59. c
60. e
61. e
62. b
63. b
64. d
65. c
66. b
67. a
68. b
69. a
70. c
71. b
72. b
73. c
74. e
75. c
76. a
77. b
78. c
79. d
80. b
81. d
82. d
83. c
84. b
85. d
86. e
87. a
88. c
89. c
90. c
91. b
92. e
93. d
94. d
95. b

96. c
97. c
98. a
99. a
100. e
101. e
102. c
103. b
104. c
105. b
106. d
107. d
108. e
109. c
110. e
111. a
112. d
113. c
114. d
115. c
116. d
117. d

Chapter 6
1. e
2. b
3. a
4. a
5. d
6. d
7. a
8. e
9. b
10. b
11. b
12. c
13. b
14. b
15. c
16. c
17. b
18. c
19. a
20. d
21. d
22. b
23. d
24. b
25. e
26. c
27. a
28. d
29. d
30. c
31. b
32. d

33. e	57. a	21. b	14. c
34. d	58. c	22. a	
35. a		23. a	**Chapter 9**
36. d	**Chapter 7**	24. a	1. a
37. b	1. d	25. b	2. c
38. c	2. e	26. c	3. a
39. b	3. c	27. a	4. d
40. b	4. a	28. a	5. e
41. d	5. b	29. c	6. e
42. b	6. c		7. d
43. c	7. a	**Chapter 8**	8. a
44. d	8. a	1. e	9. d
45. c	9. b	2. e	10. e
46. e	10. e	3. a	11. e
47. a	11. c	4. d	12. e
48. d	12. e	5. e	13. a
49. e	13. a	6. d	14. a
50. b	14. b	7. b	15. a
51. a	15. d	8. d	16. a
52. e	16. a	9. a	17. e
53. b	17. b	10. e	18. a
54. c	18. e	11. c	19. e
55. a	19. a	12. c	20. e
56. b	20. d	13. d	

Additional Resources

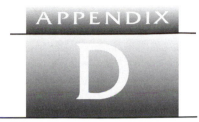

Acuson Corp
1220 Charleston Rd
PO Box 7393
Mountain View, CA 94039-7393
Phone: 650-969-9112
Fax: 650-961-2512
Toll Free: 800-422-8766
E-mail: acuson.com

Aloka
10 Fairfield Blvd
Wallingford, CT 06492
Phone: 203-269-5088
Fax: 203-269-6075
Toll Free: 800-872-5652

American Association of Physicists in Medicine
One Physics Ellipse
College Park, MD 20740
Phone: 301-209-3350
Fax: 301-209-0862
E-mail: aapm@aapm.acp.org

American College of Medical Physics
1891 Preston White Dr
Reston, VA 22091
Phone: 703-648-8966
Fax: 703-648-9176

American College of Radiology (ACR)
1891 Preston White Dr
Reston, VA 22091
Phone: 703-648-8956
Fax: 703-264-2443
Toll Free: 800-ACR-LINE

American Institute of Ultrasound in Medicine (AIUM)
14750 Sweitzer Ln, Suite 100
Laurel, MD 20707-5906
Phone: 301-498-4100
Fax: 301-498-4450
Toll Free: 800-638-5352
E-mail: membership@aium.org

American Registry of Diagnostic Medical Sonographers (ARDMS)
600 Jefferson Plaza, Suite 360
Rockville, MD 20852
Phone: 301-738-8401
Fax: 301-738-0312

American Registry of Radiologic Technologists (ARRT)
1255 Northland Dr
St Paul, MN 55120-1155
Phone: 612-687-0048
Fax: 612-687-0449

American Roentgen Ray Society
1891 Preston White Dr
Reston, VA 22091
Phone: 703-648-8992
Fax: 703-264-8863
Toll Free: 800-438-2777

ATL Ultrasound
22100 Bothell-Everett Hwy
PO Box 3003
Bothell, WA 98041-3003
Phone: 425-487-7000
Fax: 425-487-8133
Toll Free: 800-982-2011
E-mail: info@corp.atl.com

Biosound Esaote
8000 Castleway Dr
Indianapolis, IN 46250
Phone: 317-849-1793
Fax: 317-841-8616
Toll Free: 800-428-4374
Email: info@biomail.com
Diasonics Vingmed Ultrasound
2860 De La Cruz Blvd
Santa Clara, CA 95050
Phone: 408-496-3503
Fax: 408-496-3564

The Burwin Institute
120 Lake Park Dr
Winnipeg, Manitoba R2J 3A8 Canada
Phone: 204-254-1439
Fax: 204-254-7473
Toll Free: 800-322-0737
Email: burwin@fox.nstn.ca

Educational Reviews, Inc
6801 Cahaba Valley Rd
Birmingham, AL 35242
Phone: 205-991-5188
Fax: 205-995-1926
Toll Free: 800-633-4743

Educational Symposia, Inc
1527 Dale Mabry Hwy
Tampa, FL 33629-5808
Phone: 813-254-4608
Fax: 813-254-9773
Toll Free: 800-338-5901
E-mail: EDUSYMP@CYBERSPY.COM

GE Medical Systems
PO Box 414 (W-412)
Milwaukee, WI 53201
Fax: 414-544-3384
Toll Free: 800-643-6439

Hitachi Medical Corp of America
660 White Plains Rd
Tarrytown, NY 10591
Phone: 914-524-9711
Fax: 914-524-9716
Toll Free: 800-852-2080

Institute for Advanced Medical Education
14 Elm Pl
Rye, NY 10580
Phone: 914-921-5700
Fax: 914-921-6048
E-mail: INFO@IAME.COM

Medical Technology Management Institute (MTMI)
9722 W Watertown Plank Rd
PO Box 26337
Milwaukee, WI 53226-0337
Phone: 414-774-2233
Fax: 414-774-8498
Toll Free: 800-765-6864
E-mail: mtmi19@mail.idt.net

Medison America, Inc
6616 Owens Dr
Pleasanton, CA 74588
Phone: 510-463-1830
Fax: 510-463-2646
Toll Free: 800-829-7666
E-mail: marketing@medison.com

RSNA Membership Publications
2021 Spring Rd, Suite 600
Oakbrook, IL 60521
Phone: 630-571-2670
Fax: 630-571-7837

Siemens Medical Systems, Inc, Ultrasound Group
22010 SE 51st St
Issaquah, WA 98029-7002
Phone: 425-392-9180
Fax: 425-391-8362
Toll Free: 800-367-3569

Shimadzu Medical Systems
20101 S Vermont Ave
Torrance, CA 90502
Phone: 310-217-8855, ext 101
Fax: 310-217-8869
Toll Free: 800-228-1429, ext 101
E-mail: smsultrasound@cserve.com

Society of Diagnostic Medical Sonographers (SDMS)
12770 Coit Rd, Suite 508
Dallas, TX 75251
Phone: 214-239-7367
Fax: 214-239-7378
E-mail: sdms@sdms.org

Toshiba America Medical Systems, Inc
2441 Michelle Dr
Tustin, CA 92780
Fax: 714-832-3990
Toll Free: 800-421-1968

ISBN 0-07-012017-X

9 780070 120174

90000

BUSHONG: DIAGNOSTIC
ULTRASOUND